ALZHEIMER'S & DEMENTIA

Questions you have ... Answers you need

By Jennifer Hay

People's Medical Society

Allentown, Pennsylvania

The People's Medical Society is a nonprofit consumer health organization dedicated to the principles of better, more responsive and less expensive medical care. Organized in 1983, the People's Medical Society puts previously unavailable medical information into the hands of consumers so that they can make informed decisions about their own health care.

Membership in the People's Medical Society is $20 a year and includes a subscription to the *People's Medical Society Newsletter.* For information, write to the People's Medical Society, 462 Walnut Street, Allentown, PA 18102, or call 610-770-1670.

This and other People's Medical Society publications are available for quantity purchase at discount. Contact the People's Medical Society for details.

Many of the designations used by manufacturers and sellers to distinguish their products are claimed as trademarks. Where those designations appear in this book and the People's Medical Society was aware of a trademark claim, the designations have been printed in initial capital letters (e.g., Cognex).

© 1996 by the People's Medical Society
Printed in the United States of America

Library of Congress Cataloging-in-Publication Data
Hay, Jennifer, 1964–
    Alzheimer's & dementia : questions you have—answers you need
/ by Jennifer Hay.
      p. cm.
    Includes bibliographical references and index.
    ISBN 1-882606-57-4
    1. Dementia—Miscellanea. 2. Alzheimer's disease—Miscellanea.
I. People's Medical Society (U.S.) II. Title.
RC521.H39 1996
616.8'3—dc20   95-53678
                                    CIP

   3 4 5 6 7 8 9 0
First printing, March 1996

CONTENTS

INTRODUCTION

Back in the early 1960s when I was a teenager, I had a close friend whose family lived a block away from mine. After his grandfather died, his grandmother came to live with them. She was a wonderful, alert and active woman. As kids, we all enjoyed talking with her and listening to her stories of years gone by.

Not long after she moved in, we began noticing a change in her personality. It began by her repeating the same story twice, only minutes apart. When we reminded her that she had just told us that tale, she would say, "Oh, yes, I forgot." But it was more than just merely forgetting, and soon her little memory slips became more frequent. And as they increased, so did her inability even to realize that she had told us the story at all.

She also started getting confused. In the kitchen, she would ask where the chicken she had cooked the day before had gone. The fact was she had not made a chicken the day before. And when she was gently reminded of that fact, she would get angry. First her anger was self-directed. She was upset that she would get so confused. Later the anger was turned at those around her. She believed they were lying to her. Of course, she had made a chicken! Where was it hidden? Sadly, by the time she died, she did not recognize the members of her family. Physically, she had remained pretty healthy, but her mind and personality had deteriorated to almost infant levels.

Doctors in those days called her condition senility. It was attributed completely to old age. While some younger people experienced some of the symptoms, most people who suffered senility were older persons. There was hardly anything under-stood about the condition, and there was nothing that could be done to make it better.

Since then, much has changed. Researchers have discovered that not everyone exhibiting these symptoms has the same condition. In fact, there are many reasons people suffer what is now called "dementia." And dementia itself is a catchall term for a condition that manifests itself in many ways.

Probably the biggest turning point in the understanding of dementia occurred in the 1970s when the public began learning about Alzheimer's disease. This disease, which has now been identified as the leading cause of dementia, has probably been around since time began. But only in this century have researchers begun to better recognize and understand it.

Alzheimer's disease, to date, is incurable and irreversible. It has many symptoms, both cognitive and physical. And while it cannot be cured, there is much that can be done to help a person with the disease cope and adapt. Also, much can be done to help the person's family cope and adapt.

But remember that I said Alzheimer's is the *leading* cause of dementia. It is not the *only* cause. In fact, there are many people who suffer from various forms of dementia who do not have Alzheimer's disease. And there are some types of dementia that are both treatable and reversible.

Among the thousands of letters we receive at the People's Medical Society, there are many from people asking about Alzheimer's disease and dementia. These people are confused, not by the manifestation of these conditions, but by the lack of information available. They ask us for help. They want definitions, assistance in understanding the differences between the various conditions, and resources and ideas for coping.

That is why we have published this book. Jennifer Hay has researched and written a book about Alzheimer's and dementia that opens the door of understanding to all readers. It not only asks the hundreds of questions that people have, but answers them with authority and understanding.

Since first seeing my friend's grandmother suffer the effects of dementia, I have seen it more and more often. It is present in my own family, in the families of my friends, and is so commonplace that whole industries have been developed around it. Alzheimer's has become one of the most widely known diseases on the planet, a recognition of its scope and impact.

But both dementia and Alzheimer's disease are often misunderstood by a public given few answers to their many questions. This book goes a long way to curing this last condition.

Charles B. Inlander
President, People's Medical Society

ALZHEIMER'S
&
DEMENTIA

**Questions
you
have
...Answers
you
need**

Terms printed in boldface can be found in the glossary, beginning on page 173. Only the first mention of the word in the text will be boldfaced.

We have tried to use male and female pronouns in an egalitarian manner throughout the book. Any imbalance in usage has been in the interest of readability.

1 ALZHEIMER'S DISEASE AND DEMENTIA: AN OVERVIEW

Q: I've been hearing a lot about **Alzheimer's disease.** What exactly is it?

A: Alzheimer's disease is a progressive, degenerative disease that attacks the brain and impairs memory, thinking and behavior. These impairments, which can be accompanied by physical decline, lead to an inability to function normally and, ultimately, to death. In fact, Alzheimer's disease, which affects an estimated 4 million Americans, is the fourth leading cause of death among U.S. adults between the ages of 75 and 84.

Q: A person can die of Alzheimer's? I thought it was just an extreme case of **senility**!

A: It's more than that, although **dementia**—a condition that many people refer to as senility—is its most prominent characteristic.

Alzheimer's disease actually destroys brain cells. As the disease progresses, more brain cells—and more abilities—are lost. In its final stages, Alzheimer's disease affects a person's ability to control movement, bowel and bladder and his ability to communicate—leaving him completely dependent upon others, susceptible to a host of ailments and unable to recognize and seek help for his symptoms.

Q: What exactly causes death?

A: A variety of illnesses or complications—from pneumonia or heart disease to dehydration or malnutrition—may be the immediate cause, but the underlying reason is Alzheimer's disease.

Q: How long does it take for the disease to get to that stage?

A: The progression of Alzheimer's disease varies from person to person. In fact, a person can survive anywhere from 3 to 20 years after the onset of Alzheimer's symptoms, with 8 years being the average. For much of that time, he may have few, if any, physical symptoms.

Q: So what kind of symptoms *are* prominent?

A: Primarily cognitive (intellectual), emotional and behavioral ones. Alzheimer's symptoms can include gradual memory loss, a decline in the ability to perform routine tasks, disorientation, difficulty learning, the loss of language skills, impairment of judgment and changes in behavior and personality. Many of these symptoms are also symptoms of dementia.

Q: So are Alzheimer's disease and dementia the same thing?

A: They are and they aren't. Alzheimer's disease is a major cause of dementia—in fact *the* major cause—but not all dementia is the result of Alzheimer's. All people with Alzheimer's disease have dementia, but not all people with dementia have Alzheimer's.

Q: Let's back up a bit. I think I need to know a little more about dementia before we go any further. For starters, what is it?

A: Dementia is a loss of intellectual function. It includes impairment of more than one cognitive, or intellectual, ability, is persistent, is severe enough to interfere with a person's daily functioning and is often progressive, meaning it gets worse with time.

Q: So is dementia a disease?

A: Not really. Dementia is a **syndrome**—a collection of symptoms that occur together and are typical of a specific disorder or disease. In the case of dementia, those disorders and diseases—more than 70 of them in all—affect memory and/or other brain functions.

Q: Are these disorders and diseases curable?

A: Some are curable; some can't be cured but can be treated; and others can't be cured or treated. But even when no cure or treatment exists, there is much that can be done to make life better for a person with dementia.

Q: That's some consolation. Is dementia common?

A: Exact numbers are hard to come by. *Losing a Million Minds,* a 1987 government report, estimated between 2.5 million and 6.5 million people with dementia in the United States, but several factors indicate that current figures may be higher. At the time the report was published, the estimated number of Alzheimer's cases in the United States was 2.5 million. In 1989, however, a landmark Harvard Medical School study raised that estimate to 4 million—a figure substantially higher than the lower range of the 1987 government estimate for all people with dementia. In addition, the 1987 report itself predicted a 60 percent increase in the number of people with dementia by the year 2000. That 60 percent increase would place the number of people with dementia at between 4 million and 10.4 million. And the figures from the Harvard study, when coupled with Census Bureau population estimates, indicate that the number of Americans with Alzheimer's disease could reach 14 million by the middle of the twenty-first century.

So to answer your question, dementia is not only common, it is becoming increasingly more common as people live longer.

Q: Why is that?

A: Although people of all ages can suffer from dementia, the diseases and disorders that most commonly cause dementia, including Alzheimer's, affect primarily older individuals. There are, of course, exceptions. Certain diseases, such as **AIDS** and **Wilson's disease**, are more common in younger individuals, while **hydrocephalus** and brain tumors can affect people of any age. We take a detailed look at the underlying causes of dementia, who's affected and at what age in Chapters 2 and 3. For now, it's important to know that, while dementia can affect people of any age, the vast majority of people with dementia are senior citizens. In fact, dementia is the major cause of long-term disability in old age.

Q: How common is dementia among seniors?

A: Estimates vary, and exact numbers are hard to come by. But an often quoted statistic is that the incidence of dementia doubles every five years beginning at age 60. It is estimated that dementia affects 1 percent of those aged 60 to 64, 20 percent of those over 80 and more than 30 percent of those over age 85. Still other estimates, including those based on the 1989 Harvard Alzheimer's study, place the rate of dementia in people over 85 closer to 50 percent.

Whatever the actual percentages, the total number of seniors with dementia is likely to increase, since the over-65 population of the United States is expected to double by 2025.

Q: But some amount of intellectual decline is normal in old age, isn't it? Just how does dementia differ from normal aging?

A: It is true that many older people experience a minor degree of forgetfulness (known as **benign senescent forgetfulness**) as well as a slowing of physical and mental agility. In fact, the term **senile**, which many people use to mean "forgetful," is actually defined as "relating to old age."

But the forgetfulness and mental slowing that occur with age generally do not interfere with daily life; they are not disabling. Dementia, by definition, involves intellectual declines or losses severe enough to interfere with daily activities. That said, however, there is some debate among Alzheimer's researchers about whether or not Alzheimer's disease will eventually affect everyone if he or she lives long enough.

Q: You've just reminded me of another term I'm curious about. What is **senile dementia?**

A: Senile dementia is a term used to refer to dementia in people 65 and older—primarily dementias caused by progressive, degenerative diseases, such as Alzheimer's. In fact, some people still refer to Alzheimer's as senile dementia. The term **senile dementia of the Alzheimer's type** is used for older individuals who have Alzheimer's-like symptoms but whose disease has not been diagnosed with certainty. Traditionally, the term senile dementia was used to distinguish older Alzheimer's victims from those whose disease occurred earlier in life.

Q: You mean a person can get Alzheimer's before he becomes a senior citizen?

A: Yes. While the majority of people with Alzheimer's develop the disease at age 65 or older, it can strike people in their 30s, 40s and 50s. In fact, when the German doctor Alois Alzheimer first described the illness in 1906, he was documenting the symptoms of a woman in her early 50s. For much of this century, experts believed that the illness Alzheimer described—known as both Alzheimer's disease and **presenile dementia,** because it affected relatively young individuals—was different from the illness that affected primarily older individuals. Experts now believe, however, that the two diseases are the same. In other words, Alzheimer's is Alzheimer's no matter when its symptoms begin.

You may still hear the generic terms senile dementia and presenile dementia used in conjunction with Alzheimer's disease and other illnesses that cause dementia, however. They simply indicate the general age of the person experiencing dementia symptoms.

Q: While we're at this defining moment of our discussion, are there any other terms for dementia?

A: There certainly are. Terms like organic brain syndrome, chronic brain syndrome, organic mental syndrome, senile psychosis and hardening of the arteries (of the brain) have all been used to refer to dementia, as have more general terms, such as senility, brain dysfunction, cognitive impairment and mental impairment.

Q: Which terms are most commonly used today?

A: Generally, experts refer to dementia by the name of the disease or disorder that is causing it. But generic terms, such as dementia, senile dementia and presenile dementia, are used when the underlying cause is not known or when the speaker is referring to dementia in general.

Q: Speaking of dementia in general, what are its symptoms?

A: Dementia symptoms are varied and depend to a great extent on the underlying disease or disorder causing them. Not all people with Alzheimer's disease experience **hallucinations** (sensual perceptions of things that don't exist), for example, while most people with **Lewy body dementia**, an illness that resembles Alzheimer's, do hallucinate. In fact, symptoms may differ somewhat even among people with the same underlying disease or disorder. The symptoms a person develops depend in part on her underlying illness, in part on the severity and location of brain damage and in part on the person herself.

Q: I understand, but I'm still in the dark about dementia symptoms in general. What are the possibilities?

A: Dementia symptoms, like Alzheimer's symptoms, range from the cognitive to the emotional and behavioral.

COGNITIVE SYMPTOMS

Q: Can we break them down and look at each type, beginning with the cognitive symptoms?

A: Certainly. The cognitive symptoms are among the most noticeable and are often among the earliest symptoms to appear. They may include impairment, slowing or loss of:

- memory
- orientation (of time, place and people)
- insight
- logic
- judgment
- perception
- the ability to calculate
- the ability to learn new things
- the ability to use language

A person with dementia may also experience a shortened attention span and a decrease in his ability to concentrate.

These symptoms can be further complicated by perceptual problems, such as **agnosia**—the inability to associate an object with its use—and **apraxia**—the inability to use an object. There may be other types of perceptual problems, as well.

Q: Such as?

A: People with dementia may experience **delusions**—beliefs or perceptions that are untrue and incorrect. They may, for example, believe they are someone they are not. Or they may experience hallucinations—seeing or hearing things that are not there.

EMOTIONAL SYMPTOMS

Q: No wonder people with dementia often develop emotional symptoms! Are the emotional symptoms of dementia reactions to these intellectual losses?

A: In part. Just think about how you would react if, arriving at a store, you forgot what you came for. Or how would you feel if someone you didn't recognize approached you and seemed to know a lot about you? In the first instance, you might feel irritated; in the second, anxious, suspicious or even paranoid. Now imagine how you might feel if those incidents—or similar ones—occurred with regularity. Reactions to intellectual losses—or to the results of those losses—definitely affect emotions. But the emotional symptoms of dementia are not solely reactions to these types of situations. They are also rooted in actual changes in the brain.

Q: In what way?

A: The brain not only controls our thinking and physical functioning, it also controls our emotions and, ultimately, our behaviors. So changes in or damage to the brain can alter our feelings and behavior, essentially changing our personalities. As you know, Alzheimer's—and many of the other diseases and disorders that cause dementia, for that matter—destroys brain cells and damages the brain. It also alters amounts of important brain chemicals.

Q: Let me get this straight. You're saying that the emotional symptoms of dementia are caused in part by reactions to intellectual losses and in part by physical changes in the brain. Can you give me an example?

A: Certainly. **Depression** is, understandably, a common symptom of dementia. (Ironically, depression is occasionally mistaken for dementia, something we discuss further in

Chapter 2.) As you might assume, experiencing a decline in your cognitive abilities and being aware of that decline can generate emotional reactions akin to depression.

But many experts believe that the depression that occurs with dementia is also a reaction to other, physical changes that are occurring. For example, one 1995 study indicates that, at least in Alzheimer's patients, depression symptoms, such as passivity, disinterest in activity, listlessness and apathy, may actually be a result of a decrease in **dopamine**, a brain chemical—a decrease caused by Alzheimer's (*American Journal of Geriatric Psychiatry*). Regardless of whether this theory is proved true or whether it applies to people with other dementing illnesses, it illustrates the complexity of our emotions.

Q: So what are the possible emotional symptoms of dementia?

A: People with dementia may be depressed, anxious, irritable, insecure, withdrawn, afraid, hostile, jealous and/or paranoid. They may be agitated, particularly in the late afternoon or evening (a trait often referred to as **sundowning**). They may be apathetic and not react to anything going on around them (a condition known as **flatness of affect**), or they may have extremely volatile emotions, spontaneously laughing or crying for no obvious reason (a condition known as **emotional lability**). They may become stubborn and/or lose their sense of humor.

While this may seem overwhelming, remember that not everyone with dementia experiences every symptom. In addition, not every symptom a person *does* experience will continue throughout the course of her illness.

BEHAVIORAL SYMPTOMS

Q: That's good to know. Do these emotional changes have any effect on behavior?

A: Yes. The behavior of people with dementia, like that of all people, is influenced by both emotion and thought.

A person with dementia whose emotions are affected by changes in his brain may lose interest in things he once enjoyed, while a person whose dementia has affected his logical thought processes may have difficulty following through on tasks or projects. In both cases, the individual may discontinue activities that were previously normal for him, changing his typical behavior.

In addition to discontinuing normal patterns of behavior, there can also be exaggerations of existing behaviors. Behavior, as you know, is a very individual thing. That said, however, certain behaviors appear with some frequency in people with dementia.

Q: What are those behaviors?

A: Before we list them, bear in mind that not every person with dementia exhibits every behavior, and not every behavior a person *does* experience continues throughout the course of the illness that is causing dementia. We discuss the prevalence of these symptoms in more detail in Chapters 2 and 3 when we discuss the various diseases and disorders that cause dementia. For now, here are the basics.

People with dementia may experience:

- lack of initiative
- loss of interest in things they previously enjoyed
- an inability to follow through on tasks and projects
- restlessness (which can lead to wandering)
- sleep disturbances or changes in sleep patterns
- impulsiveness
- temper tantrums
- social withdrawal
- changes in attention to personal hygiene, grooming and dress

People with dementia may develop obsessive behaviors, such as repeatedly washing or rubbing their hands or rocking backward and forward. They may begin to hoard food, money or other items (although they often forget where they have hidden them). And because they are disoriented, they may get lost.

Q: Anything else?

A: As they gradually lose the socially appropriate behavior skills they learned as children, they may shed their inhibitions and begin to say or do things that would otherwise embarrass them. They may become insensitive to or inconsiderate of others or become demanding.

If their language skills are affected, their communication habits may change. They may have difficulty following a conversation, or substitute one word for another in their own speech.

If the part of the brain that controls coordination is affected, their physical coordination may decline and motor skills may suffer. They may have difficulty walking or feeding themselves; they may become incontinent.

In short, they gradually become more and more dependent on others.

Q: Some of these behaviors are frightening and dangerous. Is there any way to prevent them?

A: Many of the behavioral symptoms of dementia can be treated, regardless of the underlying cause of dementia. In fact, dealing with the behavioral symptoms of dementia is a major focus of the latter part of this book.

Q: That's good. But what about dementia symptoms overall? Are they permanent?

A: That depends on what has caused them. As we've said, some of the diseases, disorders and conditions that cause dementia can be cured, treated or held in check; others cannot. Depending on the underlying cause and the extent of brain damage, treating the illness may bring an end to dementia symptoms or at least stop them from progressing. When dementia symptoms are caused by incurable illnesses, however, they cannot be reversed.

Fortunately, even for incurable diseases such as Alzheimer's, there are measures that can be taken to treat or reduce the severity of dementia symptoms. We discuss these methods of coping with dementia in more detail later. But first, we need to take a closer look at the various diseases, conditions and disorders that cause dementia.

2 CAUSES OF REVERSIBLE DEMENTIA

Q: I want to know more about the causes of dementia. I know Alzheimer's disease is the most common cause, but I'd like to start with conditions that can be treated. If a condition can be treated, can dementia symptoms be reversed?

A: Dementia symptoms are potentially reversible in between 10 and 20 percent of people who experience them. This makes it vitally important to obtain a diagnosis as early as possible. Even treatable, curable conditions can cause irreversible dementia if they are allowed to continue unchecked. Prompt diagnosis and treatment, on the other hand, may be able to eliminate dementia symptoms or at least stop them from progressing.

Q: What are some of the conditions that produce potentially reversible dementia symptoms?

A: Drug reactions, chronic alcoholism and other types of poisoning, depression, nutritional disorders, brain disorders, diseases such as **meningitis** and **neurosyphilis**, metabolic conditions such as **hypothyroidism** and **hypoglycemia**, and problems with the functioning of the kidneys, liver, heart or lungs can all produce dementia symptoms that may be reversible.

DRUG INTOXICATION

Q: I'd like to know a little bit more about the conditions that cause reversible dementia and how they're treated. Can we start with drug reactions?

25

A: That's a good place to start—adverse drug reactions and interactions are among the most common causes of reversible dementia symptoms, particularly among the elderly.

Q: Why is that?

A: For one thing, many older people have chronic diseases and take more than one medication. (According to a widely quoted survey conducted by the Pharmaceutical Manufacturers Association, 61 percent of people over 65 take three or more prescription drugs in a given year; 37 percent take five or more, and 19 percent take seven or more.) This greatly increases their chances of experiencing adverse drug reactions and interactions. To begin with, the drugs may be incompatible with each other or with any over-the-counter medications being taken. In addition, it is possible to confuse the various drugs for one another and take them incorrectly. And the elderly are also susceptible to the standard drug reactions—like allergies and side effects—that plague everyone else, so taking multiple medications increases their chances of having reactions.

Further complicating matters is the fact that, as people age, their body weight and composition change and their livers and kidneys function less efficiently. These changes affect the way their bodies break down and use drugs, altering the appropriate dosages and making some drugs totally inappropriate. And since few studies are done on drugs' effects on older individuals, many seniors are given drugs that are inappropriate for them. In fact, according to a study reported in the July 27, 1994, *Journal of the American Medical Association,* an estimated one in four older Americans healthy enough to live at home (some 6.6 million people) is taking potentially dangerous or inappropriate medications.

Q: No wonder drug reactions are common in the elderly! Are there any specific types of drugs that pose problems?

A: There certainly are. Drugs prescribed for a wide variety of common conditions, including **hypertension** (high blood pressure), heart conditions, depression, anxiety, sleeping problems, gastrointestinal problems and **Parkinson's disease**, can cause mental impairment either alone or in combination with other drugs. Mind-affecting drugs, such as tranquilizers, **antipsychotic** medications and **antidepressants**, carry the biggest risk for mental impairment.

Some specific examples are:

- antidepressants, such as fluoxetine (Prozac), amitriptyline (Elavil) and lithium (Eskalith)

- antipsychotics, such as haloperidol (Haldol), thioridazine (Mellaril) and chlorpromazine (Thorazine)

- barbiturates, such as phenobarbital (Luminal, Solfoton) and pentobarbital (Nembutal)

- tranquilizers, such as lorazepam (Ativan), flurazepam (Dalmane), chlordiazepoxide (Librium), oxazepam (Serax), triazolam (Halcion), temazepam (Restoril), chlorazepate (Tranxene), diazepam (Valium) and alprazolam (Xanax)

Other types of drugs that can produce dementia symptoms include:

- hypertension drugs: beta blockers, such as propranolol (Inderal) and timolol (Blocadren); **diuretics**, such as methyldopa/hydrochlorothiazide (Aldoril), chlorothiazide (Diuril) and reserpine/chlorthalidone (Regroton); reserpine/hydralazine/hydrochlorothiazide (Ser-Ap-Ese); and adrenergic stimulants, such as methyldopa (Aldomet)

- heart drugs, such as digitalis and digoxin (Lanoxin)

- gastrointestinal drugs, such as cimetidine (Tagamet), famotidine (Pepcid) and ranitidine (Zantac)

- Parkinson's disease drugs, such as trihexyphenidyl (Artane), levodopa (Dopar) and carbidopa/levodopa (Sinemet)

Bear in mind that these are just examples. Other drugs of these types, as well as drugs of other types, can also produce dementia symptoms.

Q: What types of dementia symptoms can these drugs produce?

A: Drug reactions and interactions—also known as **drug intoxication**—can cause cognitive symptoms such as forgetfulness, confusion and disorientation, as well as physical symptoms such as changes in balance and gait. They can also cause delusions, hallucinations, paranoia and depression.

Q: Do these symptoms go away when a person stops taking the drug or drugs?

A: Yes, unless permanent damage has been done. Generally, if a doctor suspects that drug intoxication is causing dementia symptoms, she will remove drugs from the patient's regimen, replacing them with substitutes, if necessary, until she determines which drug or combination of drugs is responsible. Once she identifies the culprit(s), she may alter the dosage, replace the drug(s) or eliminate it (them) altogether.

ALCOHOL AND OTHER POISONS

Q: What about alcohol? That's a drug, isn't it?

A: It certainly is, and as we mentioned earlier in this chapter, chronic alcoholism can produce dementia symptoms.

Q: You can't be talking about the symptoms of alcohol intoxication, can you? They're just temporary.

A: In most instances, that's correct. The decrease in mental and physical functioning caused by occasionally excessive alcohol consumption is generally temporary. With the possible exception of a hangover, functioning usually returns to normal by the next day. But chronic alcohol abuse can produce more persistent symptoms. In fact, alcoholism is directly or indirectly responsible for more neurological disorders than any other drug, toxin or environmental agent, according to a review published in the U.S. Department of Health and Human Services' *Alcohol Health & Research World* (April 1994).

Q: Do the symptoms persist because continuous drinking prohibits alcohol's effects from wearing off?

A: That's part of the problem, to be sure. But it is not the whole story. When consumed in excess for an extended period of time, alcohol can actually damage brain tissue. In addition, alcohol abuse can lead to malnutrition. Both brain damage and malnutrition can produce dementia symptoms.

Q: Which symptoms can alcohol abuse cause?

A: In addition to the incoordination, slurred speech, balance problems and loss of inhibitions we typically equate with being intoxicated, alcohol abuse can also result in memory loss, confusion and apathy.

Q: Does abstinence reverse these symptoms?

A: Depending on the cause of the underlying problem and the extent of brain damage, abstaining from alcohol may partially reverse dementia symptoms. In many cases, including **Wernicke-Korsakoff syndrome**, a dementing illness that occurs primarily in alcoholics, treatment may also include the administration of nutritional supplements to adjust for vitamin deficiencies. Bear in mind, however, that if permanent brain damage has occurred, dementia symptoms, too, may be permanent. In that case, abstinence and nutritional supplements may succeed only in stopping the progression of those symptoms.

Q: Did you say other toxins can also cause dementia symptoms?

A: Inhalation, long-term handling, ingestion or other exposure to pesticides, industrial pollutants, heavy metals such as lead and mercury, and carbon monoxide can also cause confusion and other symptoms of dementia.

Q: Does reducing exposure reverse dementia symptoms?

A: As with alcohol, it depends on the extent of damage. In many cases, reducing exposure to the toxin or, in the case of heavy-metal poisoning, having a doctor remove it from the body using drugs that bind to the metals and escort them out of the body (a process known as chelation), can reverse dementia symptoms or at least stop their progression.

DEPRESSION

Q: Did you say depression is also a cause of reversible dementia symptoms?

A: Yes. Depression is not only a symptom of dementia, but it can cause other symptoms typical of dementia, as well. Consequently, depression is often misdiagnosed as dementia, particularly in the elderly. This misdiagnosis is tragic, because the majority of people with depression can be effectively treated.

Q: What symptoms does depression share with dementia?

A: In addition to the depressed mood, loss of interest and social withdrawal we commonly think of as depression, both syndromes can produce sleep disorders, weight loss or weight gain, **psychomotor retardation** (an abnormal slowing down of activities and mental processes) and a diminished ability to think or concentrate. In many instances, depressed people, particularly older individuals, may appear confused and may suffer memory loss.

Q: I can see how dementia and depression can be confused. How does a doctor determine which one is actually causing those symptoms?

A: We discuss diagnosis in Chapter 4. In general, however, people with dementia score differently on neurological tests and mental-status tests than people with depression. And psychological testing or psychiatric examination can offer additional information, if needed.

Q: You said that most instances of depression can be treated. How?

A: The most common methods used to treat depression are **psychotherapy**, which employs psychological methods ranging from psychoanalysis to behavioral modification, and **pharmacotherapy**, which uses antidepressant drugs. Treatment may involve either method or a combination of the two.

Q: Can these treatments be used to relieve depression in people whose dementia is caused by some other problem?

A: With some modifications, yes. Standard psychotherapy is generally effective only in the early stages of progressive, irreversible dementia, when the patient still has certain cognitive abilities intact. But modified psychotherapy, music therapy or art therapy may be helpful in later stages. And while some antidepressants can exacerbate dementia's cognitive symptoms, others can be used to improve depressive symptoms and improve function. We discuss these treatments in more detail in Chapter 5.

NUTRITIONAL DEFICIENCIES

Q: What about nutritional deficiencies? What kind of symptoms do they produce?

A: That depends on which nutrient is deficient. Different vitamins and minerals are responsible for different bodily functions and, when deficient, different symptoms. Generally speaking, the B vitamins (including B_{12}, folic acid, niacin and thiamin), which are responsible for the body's use of energy from foods and for normal tissue production, produce a variety of dementia symptoms when deficient.

Vitamin B_{12}, for instance, supports the growth and function of nerves and the spinal cord. Deficiency of this vitamin is linked to a deterioration in mental functioning, to neurological damage and to a number of psychological disturbances. The symptoms that parallel those of dementia include memory loss, disorientation, changes in personality or mood, and hallucinations.

Q: What about the other vitamins you mentioned?

A: A deficiency of folic acid, which is involved in the synthesis of nucleic acid, the genetic building block for all cells, can produce fatigue and loss of appetite. Niacin deficiency can produce irritability, anxiety, depression and other dementia symptoms; and a deficiency of thiamin, which is necessary for normal brain and nerve function, can result in depression, irritability, concentration difficulties, fatigue, lack of appetite and weight loss.

Q: Do deficiencies in any other vitamins and minerals cause dementia symptoms?

A: Yes. Vitamin E deficiency can produce lethargy, apathy, inability to concentrate and a loss of balance. And deficiencies in the minerals calcium and magnesium have also been known to cause dementia symptoms.

Q: How are these nutritional deficiencies treated?

A: Primarily by increasing a person's intake through diet, supplements or injections. Once a deficiency has been identified and corrected, symptoms generally disappear.

BRAIN DISORDERS

Q: Back at the beginning of this chapter, you said that certain brain disorders can cause reversible dementia symptoms. What kind of disorders?

A: Some brain tumors, head injuries, **subdural hematomas** (pools of blood between the brain and one of its protective membranes) and a condition known as **normal-pressure hydrocephalus** can all cause potentially reversible dementia symptoms.

Q: Brain tumors? Are you talking about cancer?

A: Yes and no. Tumors—masses or growths of abnormal cells—are either cancerous (malignant) or noncancerous (benign). Both types can occur in the brain, where they can cause such symptoms as lethargy, weakness, personality changes and intellectual deterioration.

Q: You said that the dementia symptoms caused by *some* brain tumors have the potential to be reversed. Are you referring to the benign ones?

A: Not necessarily. Although cancerous brain tumors obviously pose a threat to a person's health, even noncancerous brain tumors can be deadly. In fact, in some instances, noncancerous tumors may pose more of a threat than cancerous tumors.

Q: Why is that?

A: Because treatment for brain tumors is dependent upon the location and size of the tumor. Some tumors are easily accessible and can be surgically removed; others are not accessible and cannot be removed. It is the tumor's location—not simply whether or not it is cancerous—that determines the success of treatment.

Q: Is surgery the only possible treatment for brain tumors?

A: No. Cancerous tumors can be treated with radiation and/or chemotherapy. **Corticosteroid** drugs can be used to reduce swelling caused by either type of tumor. And in some cases where the tumor cannot be completely removed with surgery, it is possible to remove part of the tumor, relieving some pressure on the brain.

Q: Can these treatments reverse dementia symptoms?

A: In many cases, yes. But not all brain tumors can be treated successfully, so we cannot say that treatment reverses dementia symptoms in all instances. As we've indicated, brain tumors can also produce irreversible dementia.

Q: Does the same thing hold for head injuries?

A: Yes. With medical treatment, including drugs to reduce swelling, and the brain's normal healing process, some brain damage caused by head injury can be reversed, leading to a reversal of dementia symptoms. In other instances, physical, occupational or speech therapy and cognitive retraining can enable undamaged areas of the brain to assume the functions of damaged areas. But the success of these treatments depends on the location and extent of brain damage. In some instances, dementia symptoms can be reversed; in others, they cannot.

Q: **What about subdural hematomas? You said they were pools of blood in the brain. What causes them?**

A: Subdural hematomas occur when blood vessels between the brain and a membrane covering the brain rupture, allowing blood to leak out. They are usually the result of a head injury. The blood forms a mass called a **hematoma**, which compresses the brain tissue.

Q: **How is this pressure relieved?**

A: The patient may be given corticosteroid or diuretic drugs to control brain swelling. If the blood remains liquid, it may be drained in a relatively simple procedure known as evacuation; if the blood has clotted, the clot can be removed surgically.

Q: **Does normal-pressure hydrocephalus also refer to pressure on brain tissue?**

A: The pressure being referred to in this instance is that of the **cerebrospinal fluid (CSF)**, a fluid that flows through and protects the brain and spinal canal. Generally, this fluid filters through a membrane in the brain and is later reabsorbed by the spaces above the brain. Hydrocephalus, or "water on the brain," occurs when there is an interference with the normal circulation of CSF that allows excess fluid to collect in the brain. In most cases, this excess fluid is under high pressure. In normal-pressure hydrocephalus, however, the fluid pressure is normal.

Q: **What causes normal-pressure hydrocephalus?**

A: Normal-pressure hydrocephalus can be triggered by meningitis or a head injury, but in many instances, its origins are unknown.

Q: How is it treated?

A: Hydrocephalus can be treated with a surgical procedure in which a shunt—a tube, with or without valves, that carries fluid from one place to another—is implanted in the brain to circumvent any blockages and divert any excess cerebrospinal fluid.

Q: And that allows the symptoms to reverse?

A: In some instances, yes.

DISEASES

Q: You mentioned two diseases that can produce reversible dementia symptoms—meningitis and neurosyphilis. I've heard of both, but I'm a little vague on what they are. Can you refresh my memory?

A: Meningitis is an infection or swelling of the membranes that cover the brain and spinal cord. Although meningitis can be caused by bacteria or viruses, fungi or **tuberculosis** is usually responsible for the form that produces dementia symptoms. Depending on the cause of the disease, antibiotics, anti-fungal drugs or tubercular drugs are given. If the treatment is administered before permanent damage has been done, dementia symptoms may be reversed.

Q: And neurosyphilis? Is it related to syphilis?

A: It certainly is. Neurosyphilis is an infection of the central nervous system (brain and spinal cord) caused by

Treponema pallidum, the bacterium that causes syphilis. Neurosyphilis occurs in syphilis's third, final stage and was once a common cause of dementia. Its prevalence has diminished, however, with the development of antibiotics and effective methods of preventing this sexually transmitted disease. Antibiotics are extremely effective in treating syphilis in its early stages, thus preventing the development of neurosyphilis, and they are fairly effective in treating late-stage syphilis, reversing or at least halting the progression of dementia symptoms.

METABOLIC CONDITIONS

Q: **What about hypothyroidism and hypoglycemia? Again, I've heard the terms but can't quite remember what they are.**

A: Let's start with hypothyroidism. This condition occurs when the thyroid gland—the gland that regulates our metabolism—does not produce enough thyroid hormone. This can result in lethargy and a slowing of physical and mental functions. But hypothyroidism can be treated by ingesting additional thyroid hormone. This generally reverses dementia symptoms.

Q: **And hypoglycemia?**

A: Hypoglycemia occurs when the concentration of glucose (sugar) in the blood falls below normal, starving the body's cells of needed energy. Hypoglycemia can result in weakness, trembling, dizziness, confusion, difficulty walking and unusual behavior, including stubbornness and uncooperativeness. It often occurs in people with diabetes who have taken too large a dose of insulin or oral hypoglycemic medication, missed a meal or participated in extended or vigorous physical activity.

Rapidly treated by ingesting sugar, hypoglycemia is generally confused for dementia only in cases in which it occurs chronically—i.e., when diabetes is unchecked, untreated or undiagnosed.

ORGAN DYSFUNCTION

Q: **You mentioned that problems with the liver and kidneys can produce dementia symptoms. I know those organs are important, but how do they affect the brain?**

A: The liver produces bile (necessary for fat digestion) and processes glucose, proteins, vitamins and other nutrients necessary for bodily function. It also detoxifies the blood of alcohol, nicotine and other harmful substances. The kidneys also rid the body of toxins; they remove normal waste products from the blood. Dysfunction of these organs can allow toxins to circulate throughout the body and impair the processing of needed nutrients, affecting the entire body—brain included.

Q: **Can liver or kidney dysfunction be treated?**

A: That depends on the specific problem. Many liver and kidney problems, including infections, dehydration and other conditions that cause dementia symptoms, can be treated with relative ease. But serious conditions, such as those involving organ failure, may require organ transplantation to replace the organ or, in the case of kidney failure, dialysis to filter blood mechanically. In these instances, dementia symptoms are only one part of a more serious problem.

Q: **I'm a little more clear about how the heart and lungs can affect the brain. After all, the heart pumps blood and the lungs supply oxygen. But what specific problems with those organs produce dementia symptoms?**

A: As you've indicated, we're referring to chronic problems that deprive the body of needed blood and oxygen. These include **congestive heart failure**, a condition in which the heart fails to pump blood effectively, and **hypoxia**, a situation in which there is too little oxygen present in the body's cells.

Q: Can you tell me a little more about congestive heart failure?

A: Congestive heart failure generally develops over a long period of time. For one or more of a variety of reasons, the heart fails to pump blood effectively. This decreases blood flow throughout the body and causes blood to back up into the veins that return blood to the heart (hence the congestion). It can also affect the functioning of the kidneys and liver, which, as we've seen, can affect brain function.

Q: Can congestive heart failure be treated?

A: Yes. Treatment includes rest, a low-salt diet and medications such as the heart drug digitalis, diuretics (which promote urination and speed the elimination of sodium and water from the body) and **vasodilators** (which dilate the arteries, reducing the work the heart has to do and allowing it to pump blood more effectively). Depending on the cause of the problem, surgery may also be warranted.

Generally, confusion or any other dementia symptoms that accompany congestive heart failure reverse or at least stop progressing when the heart is able to pump blood more effectively.

Q: Do heart problems cause hypoxia?

A: They can. Hypoxia can also be caused by blood loss or chronic lung diseases. In hypoxia, the amount of oxygen flow to the body's cells slowly decreases, causing fatigue, slow mental responses and an inability to perform physical tasks.

Q: How is hypoxia treated?

A: Treatment may include heart- and lung-stimulating drugs or oxygen therapy. This generally reverses the above-mentioned dementia symptoms or at least stops their progression if permanent brain damage has occurred.

Q: Are there any other causes of reversible dementia?

A: Those are the major ones. That does not mean, however, that they are the only ones. Remember, more than 70 diseases, disorders and conditions can cause dementia symptoms. We tackle the most common causes of irreversible dementia in the next chapter.

3 CAUSES OF IRREVERSIBLE DEMENTIA

Q: What are the causes of irreversible dementia?

A: The most common cause is Alzheimer's disease, which may be responsible for up to 75 percent of all cases of true dementia. **Vascular dementia**, caused by problems with the blood vessels, is also a major cause. And a number of dementia cases are caused by a combination of Alzheimer's disease and vascular dementia, known as **mixed dementia**.

While these three causes account for the vast majority of irreversible dementia cases, they are by no means alone. Several relatively rare diseases can cause progressive dementia similar to Alzheimer's. In addition, there are several relatively serious conditions in which dementia may occur as a secondary manifestation of the illness.

Q: You mean there are actually diseases in which dementia is not the most prominent symptom? That's hard to believe.

A: It's hard to believe until you know which diseases and syndromes we're referring to. In fact, you may not even be aware that these conditions can cause dementia. For example, dementia can occur with Parkinson's disease and with AIDS. But those diseases produce a variety of challenging primary symptoms and are serious conditions in their own right.

When dementia does occur with these illnesses, it occurs as a secondary symptom. Secondary symptoms do not appear in all instances of a disease; primary symptoms generally do. Thus, all people with Parkinson's disease experience tremors or other movement difficulties characteristic of the disease, while only a certain percentage experience dementia. Likewise, when dementia *does* occur in one of these illnesses, it does not occur alone. The person experiencing dementia also experiences all of the other primary symptoms of the underlying disease.

Q: Okay, you've made me a believer. What are some of the other conditions for which dementia is a secondary manifestation?

A: In addition to Parkinson's and AIDS, dementia can occur in **multiple sclerosis, Huntington's disease** and Wilson's disease.

Q: I know there's no cure for AIDS and some of the other diseases you just mentioned, but some can be treated. Can these treatments reverse dementia in the diseases that cause it?

A: No. Remember, at this point in our discussion, we're dealing with irreversible dementia. True, there are treatments for some of the conditions we've mentioned. These treatments can alleviate some of the primary symptoms caused by the illness and, in some cases, stop dementia from progressing. But they cannot reverse dementia. If a person has developed dementia symptoms in the course of any of these illnesses, she will retain those symptoms. Fortunately, as we discuss in Chapters 5 and 7, there are management techniques and medications to help alleviate some dementia symptoms.

PARKINSON'S DISEASE

Q: Before we get to that point, I need to know more about what's causing those symptoms in the first place. Since you mentioned Parkinson's disease first, let's start with that. What exactly is it?

A: Parkinson's disease is a progressive disorder of the central nervous system that causes a deficiency of the **neuro-**

transmitter dopamine—a chemical necessary for transmitting messages in the brain. Its primary symptoms include tremors, stiffness in the limbs and joints, speech impediments and difficulty initiating physical movement. In later stages of the disease, however, dementia symptoms, such as memory loss, may develop.

Q: How common is Parkinson's disease?

A: Parkinson's disease affects more than 1 million Americans, causing dementia in an estimated 15 to 30 percent. In addition, for reasons not completely understood, some people with Parkinson's disease develop Alzheimer's disease and vice versa.

Q: When does Parkinson's disease usually begin?

A: Parkinson's disease usually develops in mid- to late life (after age 40) and progresses slowly for an average of 10 to 15 years, before causing disability. The majority of cases are of unknown origin.

Q: Can Parkinson's disease be treated?

A: Although there is no cure for Parkinson's disease, there are treatments, including drugs, physical therapy and surgery, that can alleviate some of the symptoms and help a person maintain mobility. Levodopa, which increases the amount of dopamine in the brain, can improve motor symptoms, such as movement and balance, while **anticholinergic drugs** and antihistamines may help reduce tremors. Brain surgery can also help relieve tremors, and physical, occupational and speech therapies may help preserve movement and counteract speech impediments. None of these treatments can correct the mental changes that occur, however.

AIDS

Q: I know a little bit about AIDS, but I didn't know it could cause dementia. How widespread is dementia in people with AIDS?

A: AIDS (acquired immune deficiency syndrome) is caused by the human immunodeficiency virus (HIV). This virus can directly infect the central nervous system, resulting in brain tumors, progressive degeneration of nerve cells and meningitis or other infections. AIDS causes dementia in approximately one-third of the people it infects.

Q: What type of dementia symptoms do people with AIDS experience?

A: People with **AIDS dementia complex** may experience a variety of symptoms. Early signs of the complex, which can occur at different times throughout the course of AIDS, include memory loss and difficulty concentrating. In later stages, confusion, distraction, delayed verbal responses, social withdrawal and clumsiness may become apparent.

Q: Do experts have any idea how HIV attacks the brain?

A: Some researchers suspect that HIV-infected cells in the brain secrete chemicals that cause a buildup of calcium in the brain. Excess calcium, in turn, can damage nerve cells. With that theory in mind, the National Institutes of Health is funding studies of **calcium channel blockers** and **NMDA receptors**, drugs that block the receptors responsible for calcium secretion in the brain, to see if they can effectively treat AIDS dementia complex.

Q: Is there anything available *now* to treat dementia in AIDS patients?

A: **Zidovudine** (also known as AZT), a drug that has been used to treat AIDS itself, may have some effect on AIDS dementia complex, according to a review in the December 15, 1994, *Journal of Acquired Immune Deficiency Syndromes.* Researchers reported a significant decline in the incidence of AIDS dementia complex since 1989, when zidovudine treatment was introduced. They speculate that the drug may be effective in slowing the development and progression of AIDS-related dementia.

MULTIPLE SCLEROSIS

Q: I thought multiple sclerosis produced only physical symptoms. How does dementia fit in?

A: While the primary manifestations of multiple sclerosis (MS) are physical, the disease actually affects the central nervous system. Multiple sclerosis destroys **myelin**—the protective covering of nerve fibers—in the brain and spinal cord, affecting numerous bodily functions, both physical and cognitive.

Q: What are the actual symptoms of MS?

A: The most common symptoms are problems with movement and coordination, sensory problems such as pain, tingling or shocking sensations, blurred or double vision, urinary incontinence, problems with mental functioning, lack of energy and fatigue.

The disease, which generally starts in early adult life (between ages 20 and 40), is episodic; symptoms last for weeks or months, then diminish or regress.

Q: What causes MS?

A: No one can say for certain. Many experts believe that a factor in the immune system may be responsible, but there are other schools of thought, as well. The risk of contracting the disease appears to be greater in people who have a relative with the disease, for example, so heredity may play a role. And because the incidence of MS is higher in the northern states than in the southern states, environmental and viral sources have not been discounted.

Q: Is there any treatment for MS?

A: Treatments vary depending on which symptoms a person experiences. Muscle spasticity, for example, can be treated with baclofen and physical therapy, while inflammation and pain may be treated with corticosteroid drugs. There is no treatment to reverse or slow the dementia symptoms associated with MS, however.

HUNTINGTON'S DISEASE

Q: What is Huntington's disease?

A: Huntington's disease (also known as **Huntington's chorea**) is an inherited, degenerative brain disease that affects both the mind and the body. The disease, which usually begins in mid-life (between the ages of 35 and 50), is characterized by irregular and involuntary movements of the limbs or facial muscles (hence the name *chorea,* from the Greek word meaning "dance"), intellectual decline, personality change, memory disturbance, slurred speech, impaired judgment and psychiatric problems.

Q: Did you say Huntington's disease is inherited?

A: Yes. Huntington's disease is an **autosomal dominant** disease; if one of a person's parents carries the gene for the disease, he has a 50 percent chance of inheriting it himself.

Q: Can Huntington's disease be treated?

A: No treatment is yet available to stop the progression of the disease or the accompanying dementia, but the movement disorders and psychiatric symptoms can be controlled with drugs. And as we said at the beginning of this discussion, management techniques and medications can help control some of the symptoms of dementia.

WILSON'S DISEASE

Q: And the final disease you mentioned—Wilson's disease. Could you tell me something about it?

A: Certainly. Wilson's disease is a rare, inherited disorder in which copper accumulates in the liver and is then released and taken up into other parts of the body. It can cause hepatitis, cirrhosis and other liver problems, and can diminish kidney function. If the metal accumulates in the brain, it can also destroy brain tissue, causing tremors, muscle rigidity, speech problems and dementia.

Q: You said Wilson's disease is rare. Whom does it usually affect?

A: Symptoms of Wilson's disease usually appear in adolescence, but the disease has occurred as early as age 5 and as late as age 50.

Q: Is there any treatment?

A: Yes. Treatment involves removing deposits of copper from the body with a drug called penicillamine, which binds with the copper, allowing it to be removed from the blood. This treatment does not cure the disease; the drug must be taken throughout life. But it can improve liver function and prevent dementia from progressing any further.

VASCULAR DEMENTIA

Q: Are those the only conditions in which dementia symptoms are secondary?

A: There is one more disease that can produce dementia as a secondary symptom. In this case, however, when dementia appears, it is the most obvious manifestation of the disease.

Q: What disease are we talking about?

A: We're talking about vascular disease—actually a group of diseases of the vascular, or blood-vessel, system, including hypertension (high blood pressure), **atherosclerosis** (a buildup of fat, cholesterol and other substances that narrows arteries) and **vasculitis** (a swelling of the blood vessels caused by any one of a number of systemic illnesses).

Vascular diseases can be serious—they can put a person at risk for serious heart and cerebrovascular problems—but they have few, if any, primary symptoms.

Q: Then how do hypertension, atherosclerosis and vasculitis affect the body?

A: Essentially, they harm blood vessels and, ultimately, affect blood flow.

Take increased blood pressure, for example. The increase means that the heart is working harder than normal to push blood through the vascular system. This puts the vessels under great strain; they may become scarred, hardened and more susceptible to atherosclerosis. Atherosclerosis, for its part, produces a buildup of materials on the artery walls, causing them to narrow. And the swelling of vasculitis also narrows arteries.

Damaged, narrowed arteries can reduce blood flow. This can make it easier for a clot or other foreign matter in the bloodstream to become lodged in an artery and actually block blood flow.

Q: I understand. But where does dementia fit in?

A: When these vascular conditions impede the flow of oxygen-rich blood to the brain, the brain's ability to function can be affected. Brain cells need oxygen to function. If they are deprived of oxygen long enough, they die, creating permanent brain damage.

Q: Wait a minute! It sounds as if you're referring to stroke. Are you?

A: By definition, yes. Stroke is a sudden loss of function of part of the brain due to an interference in the blood supply. And while we generally think of stroke's physical and communicative effects—namely paralysis and speech difficulties—it can also produce cognitive, behavioral and emotional symptoms akin to those of dementia. So yes, stroke is technically a cause of dementia. But generally, when a person suffers a major stroke, people tend to refer to her symptoms as symptoms of stroke, not as dementia. When these symptoms occur alone or without evidence of a major stroke and get progressively worse, however, they are referred to as dementia symptoms—specifically, as vascular dementia.

Q: Back up a minute. How can these symptoms occur without evidence of a major stroke?

A: Quite easily. In many cases, the symptoms are cumulative, appearing only after a number of minor strokes have occurred. This type of dementia, known as **multi-infarct dementia**, is the most common form of vascular dementia. In other instances, damage occurs in areas of the brain that do not produce the standard stroke symptoms.

Q: Could you tell me more about multi-infarct dementia?

A: Multi-infarct dementia, as we've said, is caused by a series of small strokes. These strokes leave areas of dead brain cells known as **infarcts**. When enough strokes have occurred and enough brain cells have died, a person begins to experience dementia symptoms, including memory loss (particularly of recent events), speech and language difficulties, an inability to do simple or routine tasks and an inability to recognize familiar people or objects.

Although the damage occurs over a period of time, the symptoms of multi-infarct dementia generally appear rather suddenly (when damage has hit a level in which it is noticeable) and progress in a stepwise fashion, getting worse with each subsequent stroke.

Q: What causes these strokes?

A: Multi-infarct dementia can be caused by all types of cerebrovascular diseases (that is, diseases that affect the brain and vascular system). Its most common cause, however, is recurrent **cerebral embolisms**, or blood clots, which originate in the heart or one of the carotid arteries in the neck, travel through the arteries to the brain and become lodged, blocking blood flow.

Q: You said multi-infarct dementia is the most common type of vascular dementia. What are the other types?

A: There are three other major types: **strategic infarct, lacunar state** and **Binswanger's disease**. The differences among the types depend primarily on which of the brain's blood vessels they affect. Strategic infarct dementia, for example, is caused by small infarcts that are strategically positioned in blood vessels that affect several cognitive processes, while lacunar state dementia and Binswanger's disease are caused by infarcts in small blood vessels deep in the brain.

Q: Do the symptoms vary according to type?

A: Somewhat. Depending on the vessels affected, strategic infarct can affect memory, word recall, the ability to read or to calculate, the ability to distinguish between left and right and the ability to know familiar objects or persons. Lacunar state dementia and Binswanger's disease can both cause psychomotor retardation, memory disturbances and apathy.

Q: Are these types also caused by embolisms?

A: Strategic infarct can be. But lacunar state dementia and Binswanger's disease are generally caused by the effects of hypertension on the small blood vessels of the brain. Binswanger's disease can also be caused by atherosclerosis.

Q: I know that high blood pressure can be treated. Can treatment stop the progression of vascular dementia?

A: Treating hypertension and taking other measures to reduce the risk of stroke will not reverse the symptoms of vascular dementia but may stop them from progressing. We discuss treatment for vascular dementia in more detail in Chapter 5.

ALZHEIMER'S DISEASE

Q: **Wait a minute. Didn't you say that people can get both vascular dementia and Alzheimer's disease?**

A: Yes. The combination, known as mixed dementia, is responsible for an estimated 15 to 20 percent of all cases of true dementia.

Q: **And Alzheimer's alone is responsible for still more. Isn't it time we talked about Alzheimer's disease?**

A: It certainly is. Alzheimer's disease, as we've said, is a degenerative disease of the brain. For reasons not yet completely understood, the disease slowly attacks the **neurons**, or nerve cells, in certain areas of the brain, gradually eroding cognitive ability, altering behavior and affecting a person's ability to live on his own.

Progression

Q: **You said the progression of Alzheimer's is gradual. Do its symptoms follow any pattern?**

A: Yes and no. As we said in Chapter 1, the progression of Alzheimer's disease and its symptoms vary from person to person. Some people live 20 years after being diagnosed; others die after three or four years. Likewise, some people with Alzheimer's develop symptoms that others do not or develop them at different times. This is because, while the disease does affect specific areas of the brain, the order and severity in which those areas are affected differ from person to person. One person, for example, might experience severe language deficits early in the course of the disease but still be able to function well on her own for years; another might lose functional abilities early but maintain language skills. Because of this, clinicians look at the actual systems affected in order to classify the stage of an Alzheimer's patient's disease.

Q: **But Alzheimer's is progressive. Wouldn't it be easier to simply identify early, middle and late stages?**

A: It is easier, and in fact, for the layperson, experts often do refer to three general stages—mild, moderate and severe. But, as Steven DeKosky, M.D., director of the Alzheimer's Disease Research Center and professor of psychiatry and neurology at the University of Pittsburgh, explains, this method is not precise. "There isn't a way that you can clearly say how you would differentiate mild from moderate in someone on the mild-moderate border," says DeKosky, who serves as vice chairman of the Alzheimer's Association's medical and scientific advisory board. "If you use three gross stages, you may never see changes in drug trials or treatment trials." In other words, a person who experiences certain symptoms out of the order specified in a general stage may not benefit from treatments designed to address the symptoms common to that stage. That person might, however, benefit from treatments designed to alleviate symptoms common to another stage. That is why experts identify seven clinical stages of Alzheimer's according to the systems affected by the disease.

Q: **I understand. But I don't think I need to be that precise. Could you simply identify the three general stages?**

A: Certainly. Bear in mind, however, that these stages *are* general and that the actual progression of the disease can vary. The major hallmarks of the mild stage are memory loss— particularly for recent events—and difficulty learning new information. People in the mild stage may, for example, fail to remember names, miss appointments, forget phone messages, fail to pay their bills or pay bills twice. If they are still working, they may have difficulty functioning on the job. They may find socializing difficult and begin to withdraw socially, or they may lose interest in their hobbies. And they may have difficulty calculating numbers or finding specific words.

If they recognize these problems, they may develop an elaborate system of written reminders to help them get by. Because of this, and because social skills usually remain intact in the mild stage, friends, acquaintances and even some family members may not recognize that something is wrong.

Q: What about the moderate stage?

A: As the disease progresses, difficulties become more and more obvious. People in the moderate stage may experience deficits in their remote memories as well as recent memories and other cognitive abilities. Their judgment may become poor, and their appearance may change. They may make mistakes in dressing—for example, wearing clothes that do not match—or they may appear unkempt and disheveled. Spatial disorientation becomes evident, and they may get lost. Speech difficulties may appear or get worse. People in the moderate stage may have difficulty understanding and following directions, and they may develop behavior and personality changes, such as restlessness, sleep disturbances, confusion, fear and depression.

Q: And in the severe stage?

A: In the severe stage, people with Alzheimer's fail to recognize friends and relatives and have poor memories for both recent and distant events. They become more and more dependent upon others and need continual supervision. Restlessness becomes common; delusions, hallucinations and paranoia may occur. Speech may lack fluency, and they may be unable to comprehend speech. They may forget how to perform simple tasks and, ultimately, how to move their muscles. Finally, they may become mute, immobile and incontinent.

The Mechanics

Q: And all of this occurs because something is attacking the brain's neurons? What exactly do neurons do?

A: Neurons are the messengers of the brain. They are the means by which the brain orders various parts of the body to do various things. Neurons receive messages, then pass them to neighboring neurons with the help of brain chemicals known as neurotransmitters. Damage to neurons or a lack of neurotransmitters alters the flow of information. This, in turn, alters the body's ability to respond. If, for example, the brain sends a message to the hand that it should pick up an object but the message cannot get through, the hand does not respond.

Q: I think I understand. And you said Alzheimer's disease affects certain parts of the brain. Am I correct in assuming that the death of neurons in those areas is what dictates the symptoms of Alzheimer's?

A: Yes. As you probably know, different areas of the brain are responsible for governing different bodily and mental functions. Alzheimer's disease generally attacks neurons in the regions of the brain that are responsible for thought, memory and speech. The areas most affected are the **frontal lobes** and **temporal lobes** of the **cerebral cortex** (the outer layer of the brain—an area that controls higher mental functions) and the **hippocampus** (the lower region of the brain—an area that controls emotions).

Q: What exactly happens in these areas of the brain?

A: Two significant abnormalities appear: **neurofibrillary tangles**, twisted nerve-cell fibers that appear inside neurons; and **neuritic plaques**, deposits of a sticky protein known as **beta amyloid**, surrounded by the debris of dying neurons.

Q: Are these plaques the cause or the result of neuron death?

A: That's a good question—one that researchers are currently trying to answer. Researchers do know that plaques are surrounded by the debris of dying neurons, but they are not sure if beta amyloid is the cause of the neurons' degeneration or simply a by-product of it. The protein—a starchlike fragment of a larger molecule known as **amyloid precursor protein (APP)**—appears only when APP is broken down in an abnormal way. It has been shown to destroy neurons in laboratory cultures.

Q: What about the tangles? They exist within neurons, correct?

A: Correct. The tangles exist inside neurons and may alter their ability to function.

Q: Does Alzheimer's disease cause anything else to happen in the brain?

A: Yes. In addition to developing plaques and tangles, the brain experiences a depletion of the neurotransmitter **acetylcholine**. Acetylcholine is one of a group of neurotransmitters that make up the **cholinergic system**, a system that affects memory and learning. In Alzheimer's disease, this system, along with the neurons themselves, is progressively destroyed.

Q: No wonder Alzheimer's produces the symptoms it does! It seems to affect all aspects of the brain's communication system. Do experts know why this neurotransmitter is depleted?

A: They suspect that the amount of acetylcholine diminishes because the neurons that produce it die.

Theories on Causes

Q: That leads me back to my earlier question— what causes these neurons to die?

A: Again, the answer to that question is not clear. A wide variety of theories has been proposed over the years about the cause of Alzheimer's disease. These theories include: a deficit in the cholinergic system, a deficit in a brain hormone known as **nerve growth factor (NGF)**, exposure to a viral or infectious agent, exposure to environmental toxins such as aluminum, a defect in the body's immune system, destruction caused by free radicals (unbalanced substances generated by naturally occurring oxidative reactions in the body) and genetic defects or predispositions to the disease. Several of these theories have fallen out of favor, while others continue to be researched. To date, however, the cause or causes of Alzheimer's disease remain unknown.

Q: Could we look at each of these theories?

A: Yes. Let's start with the deficit in the brain's cholinergic system. There is no question that such a deficit occurs in Alzheimer's disease. As we've said, the amount of acetylcholine in the brain decreases in Alzheimer's disease. And this neurotransmitter plays a role in memory and learning. But researchers now believe that the deficit in acetylcholine is caused by the death of the neurons that produce it rather than vice versa. So while a deficit in the cholinergic system may contribute to the symptoms of Alzheimer's, it is not a likely cause of the disease.

Q: What about nerve growth factor?

A: A relatively recent theory holds that a deficit in this brain hormone might be responsible for Alzheimer's disease. NGF normally attaches itself to a protein known as p75. In test tubes, however, this protein has been found to kill brain cells when NGF is missing. Because some studies have shown that people with Alzheimer's disease have a deficit of NGF, some experts theorize that this deficit may lead to the cell destruction of Alzheimer's disease. On the other hand, some studies have not found a deficit of nerve growth factor in the brains of people with Alzheimer's disease, so the theory remains unproved.

Q: What about the viral or infectious-agent theory?

A: This theory has its roots in the fact that several dementing illnesses are caused by viruses or other infectious agents. To date, however, researchers have no evidence that Alzheimer's is transmissible, despite efforts to determine if it is.

Q: I've heard about the aluminum theory, but I'm not sure exactly where it comes from. Could you tell me about it?

A: The theory arose in the 1970s, when researchers found high levels of aluminum in autopsied brains of Alzheimer's patients. Because aluminum was also found to cause dementia in dialysis patients who were exposed to high levels of it, some experts suspected that aluminum might be a cause of Alzheimer's disease. Since then, the theory has fallen in and out of favor several times. To date, there is no evidence that aluminum causes Alzheimer's. There is, however, speculation that aluminum does play a role in the disease process. Some theorize that Alzheimer's creates a condition that results in aluminum ions replacing iron ions, accumulating in cells and contributing to dementia.

Q: Didn't I recently read something about zinc being linked to Alzheimer's?

A: Yes. In late 1994, researchers identified a possible link between zinc and the formation of plaques in the brain. In test-tube experiments, researchers found that zinc can cause certain proteins to convert to an insoluble form that is believed to kill brain cells and accumulate and form plaques. Researchers have yet to determine if this conversion also occurs in brain tissue, however, so the theory remains unproven. It is possible, however, that zinc may play a role in the disease process.

Q: What is the background of the immune-system theory?

A: This theory stems from the inflammatory response, a process that activates the immune system to attack infections and other microscopic invaders. In some instances, something goes wrong with this process, and the immune system attacks the body's own tissues rather than infections. Defects in the inflammatory response system are responsible for a variety of diseases, including lupus erythematosus and arthritis. Some researchers speculate that defects in this system could be a cause of Alzheimer's disease, as well. This theory gained favor in 1994 when a study published in the journal *Neurology* showed that twins who took anti-inflammatory drugs were less likely to develop Alzheimer's disease than their siblings who didn't. But since the inflammatory response is actually a response to a disease process, it may not be the actual cause. The response may hold promise for treatment, however, according to DeKosky.

"We don't know how to stop plaques from forming, but we do know how to stop inflammation," DeKosky says. "If anti-inflammatory medication can suppress the inflammation of plaques, it might prove to be an effective treatment."

Q: What about the free-radical theory? Does that hold any promise for treatment?

A: The free-radical theory is based on the finding that free radicals—highly reactive, charged oxygen molecules that are constantly released into the body—have the potential to damage cells. In other words, free radicals are part of the final common pathway of cell destruction. As such, free radicals may play a role in Alzheimer's disease. But no evidence to date indicates that they are the cause. Still, researchers are looking into the role that antioxidants, including vitamin E, may play in slowing down the progression of Alzheimer's disease.

Q: That leaves us with the genetic theories. I've read a lot recently about the discovery of Alzheimer's genes, so I assume genetics is the leading theory?

A: Yes and no. There is no question that genetics plays a role in Alzheimer's disease. To date, mutations of three genes have been identified as causes of the early-onset form of Alzheimer's, and a variation of a fourth gene has been identified as a risk factor for both early-onset and late-onset disease. But not all people who develop Alzheimer's have these genes. This indicates that other factors contribute to contracting the disease.

Q: Wait a minute. Could you refresh my memory about the difference between early-onset and late-onset Alzheimer's?

A: Yes. While the vast majority of people who develop Alzheimer's develop it after they have reached 65, a small percentage develop the disease in their 40s and 50s. This early-onset form of Alzheimer's often runs in families and has long been suspected of having a genetic basis. Familial Alzheimer's, like Huntington's disease, is an autosomal dominant disease: If one of a person's parents carries the gene for the disease, the person has a 50 percent chance of inheriting it himself. The late-onset form generally occurs more sporadically. Those who develop it often have no relatives with the disease.

Q: Okay. And you said that three of the four genes discovered are associated with the early-onset form of the disease—the one that's often familial?

A: Yes. The first gene identified as a cause of Alzheimer's was located in 1991. Located on Chromosome 21, it is a mutation of the gene for amyloid precursor protein (the protein that, when broken down abnormally, creates beta amyloid). A mutation of a second gene—this one found on Chromosome 14— was discovered in 1993 and is believed to be responsible for 70 percent of early-onset cases. The third mutation, identified in 1995, is located on Chromosome 1. Experts are not yet sure exactly what the genes on Chromosomes 14 and 1 do, but both appear to be involved in the production of proteins that have similar roles.

Research is now under way to determine the exact function of these proteins and also to find out if any other genes are responsible for early-onset Alzheimer's. To further complicate the picture, some families appear to have a familial form of Alzheimer's but have none of the three genes identified thus far.

Q: **What about the fourth gene—the one that increases the risk for both early-onset and late-onset Alzheimer's?**

A: Unlike the other three genes, the fourth gene is not actually a mutation, but an **allele**, or variant. This gene, which appears on Chromosome 19, governs the production of **apolipoprotein E (ApoE)**, a substance that plays a role in the movement and distribution of cholesterol for repairing nerve cells. The gene comes in three varieties—ApoE 2, ApoE 3 and ApoE 4. People inherit a copy of one type from each parent. Thus, they end up with two copies of the gene in any number of combinations.

Q: **Is one variety or combination worse than another?**

A: Yes. Researchers at Duke University Medical Center in 1993 determined that the ApoE 4 allele increases the risk of Alzheimer's disease and can hasten its onset, while the other two varieties—ApoE 2 and ApoE 3—appear to have a protective effect.

Q: **What's the problem with ApoE 4?**

A: There are two theories: One is that the protein made by ApoE 4 either promotes the accumulation of beta amyloid (the substance found in plaques) or interferes with its removal. The other is that ApoE 4 contributes to the development of neurofibrillary tangles.

Q: How could it do that?

A: The theory is that ApoE 2 and ApoE 3 help to maintain the structure of nerve cells by binding onto a protein known as **tau**, which is found in neurofibrillary tangles. By binding onto tau, the theory goes, ApoE 2 and ApoE 3 prevent tau from forming tangles. ApoE 4, on the other hand, does not bind onto tau. This allows the protein to form the tangles that disrupt the structure and integrity of the neurons.

Q: That sounds complicated. So what's the bottom line? Just how much does ApoE 4 increase the risk for Alzheimer's disease?

A: Studies have found that people without the ApoE 4 allele have a 20 percent risk of developing Alzheimer's by the time they reach 75; people with one copy have a 60 percent chance of developing the disease, and people with two copies have a 90 percent chance of contracting Alzheimer's.

Q: Ninety percent is a pretty big risk! It sounds like this ApoE 4 gene is the key to the puzzle, doesn't it?

A: It's certainly a major part, but it's not the final piece. Although ApoE 4 definitely increases the risk of Alzheimer's disease, it does not dictate who will and who will not get the disease. Some people with two copies of ApoE 4 never get Alzheimer's, while some people with no copies of ApoE 4 do. Clearly, there are other factors involved. Perhaps another gene is involved, or environmental factors contribute to the risk. Research conducted on twins—people who share the same genes—may be able to pinpoint what these contributing factors are.

Q: This is all so confusing. It sounds like you're saying that genes play a role but don't actually dictate whether a person will get Alzheimer's. Are you?

A: Yes and no. The three genes responsible for the early-onset form of Alzheimer's can dictate whether a person gets the early-onset form of the disease. The ApoE 4 gene, however, cannot. Having one or two copies of this gene simply increases a person's risk of contracting either the early-onset or late-onset form of Alzheimer's.

Q: So what are the leading theories on the cause of Alzheimer's disease?

A: According to DeKosky, there are two leading theories— one that points us back to the plaques, the other to the tangles. The first theory is that a disruption in the metabolism of amyloid causes the disease, creating the beta amyloid present in plaques. The second is that there is an abnormality in the actual physical structure of neurons that allows them to clump together and form tangles. This disrupts the metabolism in the cell and either kills it or causes it to function incorrectly.

Q: Both of those theories seem to relate back to the theories about the role of ApoE 4, don't they?

A: They are related, certainly. Researchers are currently studying the role of ApoE 4 and debating whether beta amyloid is a cause or result of cell destruction. They are also trying to determine the role of the proteins located on Chromosomes 14 and 1, since this may help them better understand the disease. Once they have a better understanding of the disease, they will be better able to slow its progress and, ultimately, prevent it from occurring altogether.

Prevention

Q: Speaking of prevention, is there anything anyone can do now to reduce the risk of contracting Alzheimer's disease?

A: Perhaps. As we've said, a study of identical twins found that those who took anti-inflammatory drugs had a lower incidence of Alzheimer's than did their siblings; other studies have found lower rates of Alzheimer's in people with rheumatoid arthritis (who often take anti-inflammatory medications); and a study of people with Alzheimer's found that those who had taken aspirin or other **nonsteroidal anti-inflammatory drugs** for a year had better verbal and mental functioning scores than those who did not. Research is now under way to determine what role, if any, anti-inflammatory drugs can play in preventing or slowing the progression of Alzheimer's disease. At this point, however, it's too early to recommend that people take anti-inflammatory medications as an Alzheimer's preventive.

Q: Anything else?

A: Evidence is also growing that estrogen may have a protective effect against Alzheimer's. Several recent studies have found that menopausal women who have used estrogen-replacement therapy are less likely to develop Alzheimer's than women who have not used the drug, although other studies have not produced the same results. Biological research conducted on animals does suggest that estrogen improves cognitive function by preserving neurons in the hippocampus and by stimulating the production of **choline acetyltransferase**, the enzyme needed to make acetylcholine. Preliminary reports of ongoing research reported at a November 1995 meeting of the Gerontological Society of America indicate that estrogen therapy may improve the mental function of elderly women with Alzheimer's or help them respond to **tacrine**, the only drug currently approved to treat Alzheimer's. But researchers are awaiting the results of two large studies to shed more light on the subject. One of the studies is following thousands of women on estrogen to see if they develop

Alzheimer's; the other is examining estrogen replacement and Alzheimer's treatment in women who have had hysterectomies.

Q: But estrogen also has side effects. And it's clearly not an appropriate preventive measure for half the population. Is there anything else that might reduce the risk of Alzheimer's? Anything safer, like exercise?

A: You might want to try exercising your mind. Several recent studies have associated higher education with reduced risks for Alzheimer's. A study of 7,528 people reported in the April 15, 1995, *British Medical Journal* found that those with higher levels of education were less likely to develop dementia than were those with only a primary education or low-level vocational training. And an ongoing study of aging nuns conducted by researchers at the University of Kentucky is finding that the sisters, who have more education than most people and live intellectually challenging lives, live longer and with better functioning than people with less education. The percentage of nuns who suffer from dementia is lower than in the general population. And those who do develop Alzheimer's disease don't get it as early or as severely as those in the general population.

Q: It doesn't really seem like a viable preventive strategy, but you have piqued my interest. What could cause this connection between education and Alzheimer's?

A: Some experts speculate that learning stimulates neuron growth, creating a larger reserve in the brain. According to this theory, more neurons are available, so it takes longer for their destruction to produce dementia symptoms. Ironically, this "use it or lose it" theory was actually borne out by a 1995 study that found that highly educated people with Alzheimer's disease tend to experience more rapid rates of cognitive decline than those with lower levels of education. Writing in the *Journal of Geriatrics: Medical Sciences,* researchers speculate that people with higher levels of education do not display their disability until the disease is at a relatively advanced stage. Another theory holds that socioeconomic forces, such as diet and environment, may make less-educated people more susceptible to Alzheimer's.

In either event, your initial observation is correct. Education is hardly a viable preventive strategy. For one thing, the link between education and lower risk is purely observational; for another, the theory that education stimulates neuron growth has not yet been proved. And even if it is proved in the future, it's unlikely that doctors will begin writing out prescriptions for college courses or that insurers will begin distributing scholarships.

Q: **Have any other factors been observed to decrease or increase the risk of Alzheimer's disease? Anything that may help me prevent the disease?**

A: Head trauma, particularly when accompanied by a loss of consciousness, has been shown to increase the risk of Alzheimer's disease. Still, short of advising you to avoid getting hit in the head or to watch out for falling objects, there's little you can do to reduce this risk.

Q: **In other words, risk reduction and prevention strategies are still pretty much unknowns, aren't they? In fact, it seems like Alzheimer's disease involves a lot of unknowns, doesn't it?**

A: Yes. Although research is proceeding at a rapid pace, there are still many unknowns. "The rate of production of information about the disease is immense," DeKosky says. "But we have not yet reached a point where we're able to assimilate that information and put the changes that have occurred into perspective." But the race is on to do just that, since the baby-boom generation is rapidly approaching the age at which Alzheimer's becomes common. If the progression of Alzheimer's disease can be slowed by 5 or 10 years, DeKosky says, most of the people who get the disease late in life will be able to live out their lives in a relatively normal fashion, saving the nation $50 billion. "We spent the '70s and '80s looking at the pathology—the plaques and tangles and neurotransmitters. We spent the late '80s and the early '90s looking at proteins and genetics. We'll spend the next decade finding a drug," he says.

Q: Are there any other progressive, irreversible dementias like Alzheimer's?

A: There are several. Fortunately, however, none of them is common. These diseases include **Pick's disease**, Lewy body dementia and **Creutzfeldt-Jakob disease**.

PICK'S DISEASE

Q: Would you tell me more about Pick's disease?

A: Certainly. Pick's disease, which affects many of the same areas of the brain that Alzheimer's affects, is also similar in course. In fact, sometimes Pick's disease is clinically indistinguishable from Alzheimer's disease until after death. There are instances, however, where the symptoms and their progression differ from that of Alzheimer's.

In Pick's disease, for example, personality changes, blunted or excited moods or emotions, and loss of social restraints may occur early in the disease. People with Pick's may experience less disorientation than people with Alzheimer's, and memory may remain intact longer. As the disease progresses, however, behavior and language abilities deteriorate and more cognitive losses become apparent. In the final stages, patients may become mute, immobile and incontinent and may lose muscle control.

Q: You said that Pick's disease affects many of the same areas of the brain that Alzheimer's affects. Which areas, and how are they affected?

A: Pick's disease causes severe atrophy of the frontal portions of the brain's frontal and temporal lobes, which control personality, planning and judgment, smell and some aspects of memory and learning. Atrophy is also possible in other areas of the brain.

In affected areas, the neurons, or brain cells, are filled with masses of straight fibers—fibers that differ in shape and structure from those found in the brains of people with Alzheimer's. And some neurons contain densely packed, spherical deposits of protein known as **Pick bodies**.

Q: What causes Pick's disease?

A: As with Alzheimer's disease, the exact cause or causes of Pick's disease are unknown. It appears that heredity may play a role, and the disease is more prevalent among women than men. Pick's, like Alzheimer's, also appears to be related to age. The disease primarily affects people in mid- to late life.

Q: How is Pick's disease treated?

A: As with Alzheimer's disease and many of the other progressive dementias, there is no cure for Pick's disease. There are, however, management techniques and medical treatments that can alleviate some of the symptoms and improve quality of life. We discuss these methods in Chapters 5 and 7.

LEWY BODY DEMENTIA

Q: Before we get to that, I need information on the other primary dementias. Could you tell me more about Lewy body dementia?

A: Lewy body dementia is a rare, degenerative brain disease that resembles Alzheimer's disease in its symptoms and course. And, like Pick's disease, it is often misdiagnosed as a more common condition, such as Alzheimer's or vascular dementia.

People with Lewy body dementia experience confusion and attention deficits early in the course of their illness. Other symptoms include memory loss (especially for recent events), communication difficulties, agitation, hallucinations and delusions. The latter two often occur early in the course of the dementia, as opposed to later, as in Alzheimer's disease.

Initially, impairment may be mild and may fluctuate from day to day. Eventually, however, people with the disease develop severe and constant dementia.

Q: What causes this disease?

A: Again, that answer is unknown. It is known, however, that the disease is associated with protein deposits called **Lewy bodies**, which appear in deteriorating nerve cells in the brain. These deposits, which can also be found in the brains of people with Parkinson's disease, cause dementia symptoms when they are found in the brain's outer layer—the cerebral cortex. This part of the brain controls higher mental functions, including speech and language, movement and behavioral reactions.

CREUTZFELDT-JAKOB DISEASE

Q: I'd like to know more about Creutzfeldt-Jakob disease. What is it and how does it affect people?

A: Creutzfeldt-Jakob disease is a fatal brain disorder that causes dementia and a variety of other neurological symptoms. In its early stages, it produces memory losses, behavioral changes, incoordination and visual disturbances. As it progresses, mental deterioration becomes more pronounced, jerks and other involuntary movements develop, and blindness and weakness may develop. Ultimately, the patient falls into a coma and dies. This can occur within a year of the onset of symptoms.

Q: That's fast! Is this a common disease?

A: Fortunately, no. In fact, since the disease was identified in the 1920s, only in excess of 3,000 cases have been reported worldwide. The disease is more prevalent in certain areas, such as rural Slovakia and Chile. In the United States, it affects and kills an estimated 200 people each year. Unfortunately, however,

Creutzfeldt-Jakob can be transmitted from one person to another and can affect virtually anyone.

Q: Why? What causes this disease?

A: Creutzfeldt-Jakob disease is caused by an unknown organism—possibly a "slow" or "unconventional" virus. The organism appears to have a very long incubation period; it can take three years or longer before symptoms first appear. And it is considered unconventional because a core of nucleic acids commonly seen in other viruses has not been identified.

Q: How is this virus or organism transmitted?

A: The various means by which the virus can be transmitted are unknown. There is evidence that the disease can be introduced into the body during certain medical procedures, although this cannot account for all incidence of the disease.

Q: What kind of medical procedures?

A: According to the National Institutes of Health's Office of Scientific and Health Reports, Creutzfeldt-Jakob has been transmitted through transplanted corneas. In addition, there have been several documented cases in people undergoing neurosurgery.

Q: How else might the disease be spread?

A: In several instances, the disease has occurred in health workers who might have been exposed to the disease during the course of their work. And while the low incidence of the disease indicates that the disease is not highly contagious, person-to-person transmission may occur.

Q: Am I right in assuming there is no treatment for Creutzfeldt-Jakob disease?

A: Yes. Until researchers isolate the agent that causes the disease, a disease-specific cure or treatment is unlikely. As we've said, however, there are management techniques and treatments that can alleviate some of the symptoms. We discuss those treatments in Chapters 5 and 7, but first we need to learn how these diseases are diagnosed.

4 DIAGNOSING DEMENTIA

Q: How important is it to determine what is causing dementia symptoms?

A: Very. After all, dementia is reversible 10 to 20 percent of the time, and its progression can be slowed or stopped in other instances. Even when dementia is irreversible, diagnosis is an important first step in preparing to live with it.

Q: How do doctors determine the cause of dementia?

A: Diagnosing what is causing dementia symptoms is primarily a process of elimination. Because symptoms for many of the diseases that cause dementia are similar and there are no specific tests for some of those diseases, doctors must eliminate the various possibilities with a succession of examinations and tests.

Q: How long does the testing last?

A: That depends on how quickly the doctor zeros in on a cause. Drug reactions, which may be discovered during a doctor-patient interview, or nutritional deficiencies, which can show up in blood tests, may be diagnosed in one or two office visits, for example. In other cases, a diagnosis of Alzheimer's disease may not be confirmed until after death. Thus, the time it takes a doctor to determine what is causing dementia symptoms and the number of tests involved varies from person to person and from doctor to doctor.

Doctors who are experienced in treating dementia may be able to make a diagnosis quickly and accurately with minimal testing, while doctors who have little experience with dementia may need to run numerous tests. In any event, the primary goal of diagnosis is to determine as quickly as possible whether the dementia is treatable or not.

Q: That makes sense. Is there a standard starting point for this diagnostic process of elimination?

A: Yes. The doctor generally begins by physically examining the patient and taking a medical history.

PHYSICAL EXAMINATION

Q: What is he looking for?

A: Primarily information about the patient's current health status and symptoms. In a physical exam, for example, the doctor will take the patient's blood pressure and pulse and check her heart and lungs. He'll also ask about nutrition and diet. Essentially, he wants to know if the patient is exhibiting any physical symptoms that could give him a clue about the cause of her dementia symptoms. High blood pressure, for example, might indicate vascular dementia, while a fever might indicate an infection.

MEDICAL HISTORY

Q: What about the medical history? What is the doctor looking for there?

A: For starters, the doctor needs to know what prompted the person to come in for an examination: Remember, some dementia symptoms are more common in one disease than another, and the progression of symptoms varies according to the illness. With that in mind, the doctor needs to know exactly what

symptoms the patient is experiencing, when they began, if they
have progressed and, if they have, in what manner.

Because the patient may be unable to recognize her symptoms
or may be unable or unwilling to answer the doctor's questions,
the doctor may also ask a family member or close friend for this
information and any other information he may need to know.

Q: What else does the doctor need to know?

A: The doctor needs information about any other symptoms
or conditions the patient has recently experienced and
any drugs she has been taking: Has she had a fever? Has she com-
plained of aches or pains? Has she recently experienced a blow
to the head? Has she been taking any medications? Have any of
her medications changed recently? He'll ask many questions of
this type.

He also needs to know the medical history of the patient's
family. As we've seen, several of the diseases that cause dementia
have genetic origins, so it is important for the doctor to know
if other members of the patient's family have experienced
dementia symptoms.

NEUROLOGICAL TESTS

Q: I assume some type of testing is needed at
this point?

A: Generally. After the doctor has physically examined the
patient and taken her medical history, he'll probably want
to observe for himself the various cognitive symptoms she is exhibiting and check her for signs of other neurological problems.
After all, some of the illnesses that cause dementia also cause
problems with balance, gait, movement and other neurological
functions. These functions, along with cognitive functions, can be
evaluated with a series of brief neurological tests and a mental-
status exam.

Q: Neurological tests? What are they?

A: Neurological tests are noninvasive tests that measure bodily functions and abilities, such as reflexes, sensation, coordination, senses, language skills, balance, walking and coordination. These abilities are governed by the nervous system, a complex system of nerve cells (in the nerves, spinal cord and brain) that controls all functions of the body.

Q: What do these tests entail?

A: That depends on which abilities and functions the doctor is trying to measure. If he is trying to measure reflexes or sensation, for example, he may tap the patient's knee gently with a hammer or test her ability to feel heat, cold, pinpricks and other sensations. To test sense of balance and walking ability, he may ask the patient to stand up and walk, so he can observe her gait. And to test her strength and coordination, he may ask her to perform simple physical tasks, like putting her finger to her nose.

Q: You said the doctor may also conduct a mental-status exam. What can that tell him?

A: A mental-status exam—primarily a series of questions— is used to assess mental functions, such as memory, orientation (of people, time and place), attention, reasoning, language and the ability to follow instructions.

Q: Can you give me some sample examples?

A: If the doctor wants to know about the patient's orientation, he may ask her her name, the date or where she is. If he wants to know about her recall of general information, he may ask her who is president or how many days are in a week. If he wants to test her memory and learning skills, he may give her a list of words and ask her to repeat them later on in the test. To test her memory and attention span, he may ask her to recite the months of the year backward and forward, or to remember and repeat a series of numbers backward and forward. To test her abstract reasoning ability, he may ask her to explain something. And to test her language skills, he may ask her to name objects or demonstrate her ability to read, write and understand written language.

Q: What exactly do the results of these tests tell the doctor?

A: The results indicate which specific abilities are affected and to what extent. Remember, different dementing illnesses cause different symptoms and they progress in different ways. Knowing exactly what a person can and cannot do is a major part of determining what disease might be causing dementia.

Q: How long does all this neurological testing take?

A: That depends on the doctor and the tests he decides to use. Many of the neurological tests and standard mental exams take only minutes. The doctor may administer these tests and obtain the results he needs during the initial office visit, or he may determine that additional testing is needed and schedule a block of several hours in which to conduct more in-depth **neuropsychological tests**.

Q: Will the doctor conduct those additional tests himself?

A: He might, or he might refer his patient to a **neurologist** (an M.D. or D.O. who specializes in diagnosing and treating disorders of the nervous system), a psychiatrist (an M.D. or D.O. who specializes in diagnosing and treating mental or psychiatric disorders) or a psychologist (a mental-health professional with a doctoral degree in psychology and training in counseling, psychotherapy and psychological testing).

Whoever is doing the testing will use standardized tests to assess intelligence, memory, language and prior academic achievements. Scores on these tests can be compared with the scores of other people in the same age-group. This helps the doctor determine whether the changes in a person's mental status are caused by normal aging or by disease.

These tests—along with mental-status tests and psychological tests—also help the doctor distinguish between dementia and depression. Generally speaking, depressed people perform better than people with dementia on memory tests and are more likely to admit not knowing an answer rather than make up responses to conceal their problem.

LABORATORY TESTS

Q: **What if the results of these neuropsychological tests don't point to depression or normal aging but instead suggest that some disease or condition is causing dementia? Are there more tests that can be run?**

A: Yes. As we said earlier, diagnosing the cause of dementia is essentially a process of elimination. Once a doctor has examined a patient, learned her medical history and observed for himself her symptoms or lack thereof, he can begin to narrow down the possible causes of her problem. In most cases, he will start with a series of standard laboratory tests.

Q: **What kind of laboratory tests?**

A: The laboratory tests range from standard blood and urine tests to tests for syphilis and AIDS—diseases that can cause secondary dementia.

Q: I understand the purpose of the disease-specific tests, but what is the purpose of blood and urine tests?

A: Both blood and urine can reveal a lot about a person, including how well her kidneys are functioning and whether or not she is obtaining and metabolizing necessary vitamins, minerals and other nutrients. As you recall, kidney dysfunction and nutritional deficiencies can cause dementia symptoms.

Q: What can blood alone reveal?

A: Blood can reveal whether or not a person is fighting an infection or is experiencing liver or thyroid dysfunction. It can also be used to measure the level of glucose in the blood. Remember, certain infections—like meningitis—as well as liver dysfunction, hypothyroidism and hypoglycemia are among the causes of dementia symptoms.

Q: Are any other laboratory tests performed?

A: If the doctor suspects that heart or lung disease is responsible for the dementia symptoms, he may order an **electrocardiogram (EKG)** or a chest x-ray. An EKG measures the pattern of electrical impulses generated in the heart and can help identify damage to heart muscle, irregular heart rhythms, enlargement of a heart chamber or damage caused by a heart attack; a chest x-ray can give him a view of the lungs.

If he suspects meningitis, multiple sclerosis, a brain tumor or hydrocephalus as the cause, he may order a **lumbar puncture**. This test, also known as a *spinal tap*, involves the insertion of a thin, hollow needle into the lower back to measure the pressure of cerebrospinal fluid and obtain a sample for analysis. The pressure reading may assist the doctor in diagnosing hydrocephalus, while the fluid itself can help him determine if the patient has meningitis, multiple sclerosis or a brain tumor.

The fluid analysis may one day also assist doctors in diagnosing Alzheimer's disease. Research is currently under way on a method to measure levels of the protein tau in cerebrospinal fluid. As you may recall, tau is the protein that forms the building block of neurofibrillary tangles. Tau is present in high levels in the cerebrospinal fluid of people with Alzheimer's disease; however, it is also present at similar levels in some people who do not have the disease.

BRAIN IMAGING AND FUNCTION TESTS

Q: Those laboratory tests reveal a lot. But what if they tell the doctor only what's *not* causing the dementia symptoms?

A: If the doctor suspects that vascular dementia or a brain disorder is a possible cause, he may elect to run one or more tests to view the brain and see how it is functioning.

Q: Such as?

A: Such as **electroencephalography (EEG)**, which shows the brain's electrical activity, or any of a number of imaging tests that enable him to view the brain's anatomy and functioning.

Q: I'd like to know a little bit more about those tests. For example, how does EEG work?

A: Brain cells communicate by means of electrical impulses. Electroencephalography uses electrodes placed on the scalp to collect those impulses. If brain cells are damaged and can no longer communicate, fewer total impulses are sent, so fewer impulses are picked up by the electrodes. This would indicate brain damage—and brain damage, as we've seen, can cause dementia symptoms. But while EEG can indicate whether brain damage has occurred, it does not identify the cause of the brain damage. Its value, therefore, is limited.

Q: How about the imaging tests? What do they indicate?

A: That depends on the test. **Computerized tomography (CT)**, also called **computerized axial tomography (CAT)**, and **magnetic resonance imaging (MRI)** provide detailed images of internal body parts—in this case, the brain—while **positron emission tomography (PET)** and **single photon emission computed tomography (SPECT)** provide a picture of how those body parts and systems are working, or functioning.

Q: How do these tests work?

A: CT uses computer and x-ray technology to generate detailed pictures, while MRI uses magnetic fields and radio-frequency pulses to obtain computer-generated images. PET and SPECT are a little more high-tech. These tests create computer-generated x-ray images of the brain that track harmless **radioactive isotopes** injected or inhaled into the body. The major difference between these two tests, technically, is the type of isotope they use. The other difference is in cost: PET is much more expensive than SPECT.

Q: What can imaging tests reveal?

A: CT and MRI can reveal tumors, infarcts (areas of dead tissue), brain injuries and other areas of brain damage. They may confirm, for example, that stroke has occurred or that some other form of vascular dementia is causing symptoms. These two imaging tests are also helpful in diagnosing normal-pressure hydrocephalus, since the condition causes certain areas of the brain to enlarge. Likewise, the tests can be used to measure atrophy and deterioration of the brain, although this measurement is more useful for showing patterns and stages of dementia progression than it is for diagnosing a dementing illness.

PET and SPECT can show how the brain is using oxygen and glucose and how blood is flowing through the brain. This information can indicate whether the brain's normal functioning—its "vital signs," so to speak—has been affected and identify areas of brain damage. These tests hold some promise for diagnosing dementing illnesses in the future. At the present time, however, cost, limited availability and a lack of specificity make them more an object of research than actual diagnostic tools. (Specificity refers to the ability of a test to correctly identify those people who do not have a disease.)

Q: **Do any of these imaging tests show Pick bodies, Lewy bodies or the plaques and tangles that appear in the brains of people with Alzheimer's?**

A: Unfortunately, those characteristic signs—signs crucial to diagnosis—can be observed only in brain tissue, and brain tissue is typically not examined until after a person has died. Imaging tests can, however, show decreases in brain size and indicate the precise location and extent of brain damage. They are useful for identifying tumors, head injuries, subdural hematomas, infarcts and hemorrhages. They are not useful for diagnosing Alzheimer's disease, Pick's disease or other degenerative brain diseases.

Q: **Then how are those diseases diagnosed?**

A: These diseases can be diagnosed with certainty only after an examination of brain tissue—and this is not a common, simple test.

Remember, dementia diagnosis is a diagnosis of exclusion. If, after extensive testing, the doctor has ruled out all potentially reversible causes of dementia and all of the diseases that can cause dementia as a secondary condition, he may still be left with several possibilities, including Alzheimer's disease, Pick's disease and Lewy body dementia. In this instance, he may offer a diagnosis of dementia, senile dementia or presenile dementia and continue to observe the patient. Often, simply observing the patient as she progresses through the various stages of her illness helps him make a more definite diagnosis.

Q: What if the doctor suspects a certain disease?

A: If the doctor suspects Alzheimer's—the most common cause of dementia—he may offer a diagnosis of senile dementia of the Alzheimer's type, possible Alzheimer's or probable Alzheimer's. Similar "possible" and "probable" diagnoses are possible for progressive, degenerative dementias like Pick's disease and Lewy body dementia. While neurologists and other doctors familiar with dementia may be able to diagnose Alzheimer's disease and other progressive degenerative brain diseases with 90 percent accuracy, as we've said, the only way these diagnoses can be confirmed is by an examination of brain tissue.

Q: When is brain tissue examined?

A: Although brain tissue can be obtained through a biopsy of a live person, most doctors believe brain biopsy is an inappropriate procedure for routine diagnosis of diseases like Alzheimer's. For one thing, the operation is both expensive and potentially dangerous. For another, none of these degenerative brain diseases is curable. And the methods of managing symptoms is similar for all three. Thus, brain tissue is generally examined at autopsy—after a person has died.

Q: I read something recently about a new test for Alzheimer's disease that uses eyedrops. Has that been made available yet?

A: Several tests for Alzheimer's—including one using eyedrops—have been proposed in recent years, but as yet no effective test has been made available.

Researchers in 1994 reported that people with Alzheimer's disease appear to be extremely sensitive to **tropicamide**—a drug that dilates the pupils of the eye by blocking the action of acetylcholine. Their study, which has not yet been independently confirmed, found that the pupils of people with Alzheimer's dilated in response to a solution of tropicamide one-hundredth the strength normally needed for dilation. Until these findings are confirmed, however, this method of testing will not be available.

Q: What other tests have been proposed?

A: As we discussed earlier in this chapter, a test to measure the level of tau in cerebrospinal fluid shows promise, but it is complicated by the fact that some people who do not have Alzheimer's disease have high levels of tau in their cerebrospinal fluid.

Blood tests have also been developed to identify the variants of ApoE a person is carrying. But the presence of ApoE 4 indicates only increased risk for Alzheimer's disease. It cannot indicate whether a person will actually develop the disease, and it cannot diagnose it. Thus, the test holds little merit for the general population. A positive test result might worry people needlessly, while a negative result might give them a false sense of security.

Q: Doesn't this lack of effective testing procedures for Alzheimer's disease present a problem?

A: Fortunately, the need to obtain an exact diagnosis for Alzheimer's disease and other irreversible dementias is less pressing than the need to obtain an exact diagnosis for reversible dementia. This will change, of course, when researchers pinpoint the cause of Alzheimer's and other irreversible dementias and develop effective treatments. By that time, diagnosis may be more precise. In the meantime, however, the treatment and management of most irreversible dementias, which consists primarily of treating individual dementia symptoms, is very similar. We discuss the medical treatments in the next chapter.

5 MEDICAL TREATMENT

Q: I know treatment for irreversible dementia is limited, but I'd like to know more about it. What can you tell me?

A: There's one drug that can alleviate cognitive symptoms in some people with Alzheimer's disease. And there are drugs that control hypertension and reduce the risk of strokes in people with vascular dementia. But most of the medical treatments for dementia are designed to alleviate or reduce the effect of emotional and behavioral symptoms and improve the quality of life for people with dementia and their families. These medications play a major role in dementia treatment, and we discuss them in detail later in this chapter. But first we need to look at the medications available to treat vascular dementia and the medications being used and studied for the treatment of Alzheimer's disease.

TREATMENTS FOR VASCULAR DEMENTIA

Q: Didn't you say in Chapter 3 that treatment can actually slow the progression of vascular dementia?

A: Yes. Vascular dementia is not caused by a progressive, degenerative illness. It occurs when vascular disease permanently damages the brain. If vascular diseases, such as hypertension and cerebrovascular disease, are treated, thereby helping to prevent additional brain damage, vascular dementia may not progress at all. If treatment does not actually prevent additional brain damage but slows its onset, vascular dementia may be slowed as well.

84

Q: So how is vascular dementia treated?

A: That depends on the underlying vascular disease. For example, if hypertension is causing the problem (as it often does in lacunar state dementia and Binswanger's disease), treatment for vascular dementia will include treatment for hypertension.

Q: How is hypertension treated?

A: With lifestyle changes, medications or a combination of the two.

Q: What kind of lifestyle changes might help lower blood pressure?

A: People with mild hypertension may lower their blood pressures by increasing physical activity, limiting alcohol consumption, maintaining appropriate weight and reducing sodium in their diets. If these changes don't work by themselves, they may be recommended in conjunction with an antihypertensive medication.

Q: Is there more than one kind of antihypertensive medication?

A: Yes. There are several major classes of antihypertensives, each of which works in a different way. Diuretics, for example, rid the body of excess sodium and fluids, while beta blockers slow the heart rate and reduce the production of an enzyme that increases the blood vessels' resistance to blood flow. Other classes of antihypertensives include sympathetic nerve inhibitors, which block the brain's message to constrict the blood vessels; vasodilators, which relax the artery walls; angiotensin converting enzyme (ACE) inhibitors, which interfere with constriction; and calcium antagonists, or calcium channel blockers, which reduce the heart rate and relax blood vessels.

Q: So treating hypertension can have an effect on lacunar state dementia and Binswanger's disease. Does it have an effect on the most common type of vascular dementia—multi-infarct dementia—as well?

A: Yes, it does. After all, hypertension is a strong risk factor for stroke, and multi-infarct dementia is caused by stroke.

Q: Is treating hypertension the only way to treat multi-infarct dementia?

A: No. People with multi-infarct dementia are often treated with **platelet inhibitors**, drugs known as "blood thinners," which reduce the risk of embolism development. The most commonly prescribed platelet inhibitor is aspirin. For those who have difficulty taking aspirin, **ticlopidine**, another platelet inhibitor, may be prescribed.

Another type of blood-thinning drug used to prevent stroke is the **anticoagulant**. Because this type of drug can increase the chance of bleeding in the brain, it is generally given only to people in whom the source of the infarct has been located and who are at low risk for hemorrhage.

Q: Are there any other drugs used to treat vascular dementia?

A: We mentioned vasodilators in our discussion of antihypertensive drugs, but these drugs have also been given to nonhypertensive people with vascular dementia. In fact, vasodilators were common treatments in the past, when many doctors believed senile dementia was caused by a "hardening of the arteries."

These drugs, like papaverine hydrochloride (Pavabid), relax the heart muscle and cause the blood vessels in the brain to dilate, increasing blood flow to the brain. These drugs appear to improve sociability, alertness and mood in some people with vascular dementia, but their effects are small.

Q: Is there anything else?

A: A drug known as ergoloid mesylates **(Hydergine)** has also been used to treat people with vascular dementia, Alzheimer's disease and other progressive illnesses.

Hydergine is a **nootropic** drug—a drug whose mechanisms experts do not understand. According to the *Physician's Desk Reference,* Hydergine has produced modest changes in mental alertness, confusion, recent memory, orientation, emotional lability, self-care, depression, anxiety, fears and sociability in some people. Those who appear to be helped by the drug either suffer from an ill-defined process relating to aging or have some underlying dementing condition like Alzheimer's disease or multi-infarct dementia.

An analysis of studies on Hydergine, reported in the August 1994 *Archives of Neurology,* found that Hydergine is more effective than an inactive, or placebo, drug for treating people with dementia; generally, people with vascular dementia who were given Hydergine saw the greatest effects from the drug, while people with Alzheimer's disease saw only modest effects. Still, the American Psychiatric Association may recommend further study of Hydergine in its treatment guidelines for Alzheimer's disease, according to the October 15, 1995, *Internal Medicine News.*

TREATMENT FOR ALZHEIMER'S DISEASE

Q: That effectively brings us to treatments for Alzheimer's disease. Didn't you say there is only one approved treatment?

A: Yes. To date, the only approved treatment specifically for Alzheimer's disease is tetrahydroaminoacridine, more commonly known as tacrine, which is sold under the brand name Cognex. Approved by the Food and Drug Administration in 1993, tacrine is a palliative treatment for Alzheimer's disease—that is, it is designed to lessen symptoms; it is not designed to cure the disease itself.

Q: What symptoms does tacrine address?

A: Tacrine is designed to improve cognitive abilities, such as memory and learning. It does this by increasing the amount of acetylcholine in the brain. As you'll recall, the amount of acetylcholine, a neurotransmitter involved in memory and learning, decreases in people with Alzheimer's. Tacrine stops **acetylcholinesterase**, an enzyme, from breaking down acetylcholine.

Q: How effective is tacrine?

A: Tacrine improves cognition significantly in some people; in others, however, its effectiveness is either marginal or marred by side effects. A large study sponsored by the National Institute on Aging found that 27 percent of the people who were able to take a high dose of tacrine showed improvement on cognitive tests equal to the usual decline that Alzheimer's disease causes in a year. In another study, tacrine resulted in an eight-month improvement. But many people cannot tolerate the drug, which can cause nausea, vomiting, diarrhea and, in some cases, liver damage.

Q: In other words, tacrine isn't the treatment everybody is looking for, is it?

A: No. While 20 percent of people who take tacrine see significant improvement, others cannot tolerate the drug. Still, it offers people with Alzheimer's disease some hope for improvement.

On the Horizon

Q: Are any other drugs being studied?

A: Yes. Numerous drugs have been and are being studied for their ability either to improve the conditions of people with Alzheimer's or to slow the disease's progression. These include:

- **cholinergic drugs**
- drugs that slow or stop the degeneration of neurons
- nerve growth factor
- anti-inflammatory drugs

Cholinergic Drugs

Q: What are cholinergic drugs?

A: Cholinergic drugs are drugs that affect the cholinergic system, the system of neurotransmitters related to memory and learning. These drugs, like tacrine, are designed to increase the amount of acetylcholine.

Q: Do they work in the same way as tacrine?

A: Most do. Initial efforts to stimulate the cholinergic system focused on trying to get the body to produce more acetylcholine by giving it more choline or lecithin—precursors of acetylcholine that are found in some foods, such as eggs and soybeans, or are sold in supplement form. Unfortunately, this type of treatment did not produce the desired effects.

Researchers found more success when they turned their attention to methods to prevent the destruction of acetylcholine—drugs that, like tacrine, inhibit acetylcholinesterase. A number of these drugs are currently being studied, including **physostigmine**

(Synapton), ENA 713 and numerous other drugs with similar numerical names. Another drug that may enhance the cholinergic system is xanomeline, which selectively stimulates neurons and enhances cholinergic transmission. This drug also seems to alter the breakdown of amyloid precursor protein and could, thereby, decrease the formation of plaques. Bear in mind, however, that while cholinergic drugs do increase the amount of acetylcholine, they do not correct the reason the substance is missing in the first place—the death of the neurons that produce acetylcholine.

Drugs That Slow Neuron Degeneration

Q: Is that the job of the drugs designed to slow or stop the degeneration of neurons?

A: Yes. These drugs address various stages of nerve-cell death, including (1) a decline in the neuron's ability to carry out routine energy production and repair operations (in other words, its ability to function), (2) injuries from free radicals and (3) the disruption of the normal balance of calcium between the inside and outside of nerve cells.
  Among the drugs being studied are:

  • drugs that improve neuron function
  • antioxidants
  • calcium channel blockers

Q: What type of drug can improve neuron function?

A: Researchers are currently studying the effects of a drug known as propentofylline, which enhances blood flow and energy metabolism in the brain and may protect and improve the function of neurons. If it is proved to be effective, this drug could slow progression of Alzheimer's and improve some symptoms.

Q. Could you tell me something about antioxidants? Aren't they in vitamins?

A. Antioxidants are molecules that neutralize free radicals in the body. Theoretically, this prevents cellular damage.

Free radicals, as we discussed in Chapter 3, are unstable molecular fragments naturally produced in the body during reactions involving oxygen. Free radicals damage cells—including nerve cells. And yes, a number of vitamins, including vitamins C and E and beta-carotene, are antioxidants.

Q. So are we talking about treating Alzheimer's disease with vitamins?

A. Not exactly, although vitamin E is being studied in conjunction with a drug called **deprenyl**, which is used to slow the progression of Parkinson's. Deprenyl is being studied because autopsies of the brains of people with Alzheimer's disease show elevated levels of monoamine oxidase, and deprenyl is a monamine oxidase inhibitor with antioxidant properties.

Researchers are also studying an extract made from the leaves of the *Ginkgo biloba* tree. This extract, which appears to increase circulation in the brain and act as an antioxidant, was found in a 1994 study to improve memory in people in the early stages of Alzheimer's disease.

Q. And calcium channel blockers? I thought you said they were used to treat hypertension.

A. They are. But a common theory holds that an imbalance of calcium inside and outside neurons can lead to their destruction. With that theory in mind, researchers are currently studying whether the calcium channel blocker nimodipine can prevent that imbalance from occurring by preventing calcium from entering neurons.

Nerve Growth Factor

Q: Did you say researchers are also studying nerve growth factor?

A: Yes. As we said in Chapter 3, some experts theorize that a deficit in nerve growth factor (NGF) plays a role in Alzheimer's disease. This brain hormone, which stimulates the growth of cholinergic neurons, has been shown in several small European trials to improve memory and thinking in several individuals with Alzheimer's disease. But a major hurdle must be overcome before it can be tested widely: NGF is too large to pass through the blood-brain barrier. The only way to get the hormone into the brain is by drilling a hole in a person's skull. Until a better method is found to get nerve growth factor into the brain, it is unlikely that it will be commonly used to treat Alzheimer's disease.

Anti-Inflammatory Drugs

Q: That's certainly logical. At least anti-inflammatory drugs are a little bit easier to administer. Which drugs are being studied?

A: As we saw in Chapter 3, evidence from several studies indicates that anti-inflammatory drugs might reduce the risk of Alzheimer's disease. As a result, researchers are currently investigating whether the drugs might have value in treating the disease. Some initial results look promising.

Research published in *Neurology* in August 1993 found that Alzheimer's patients' performance on cognitive tests improved 1.3 percent if they took **indomethacin** (Indocin), a nonsteroidal anti-inflammatory drug, for six months, and declined 8.4 percent if they took a placebo. And a small study reported in the January 1995 issue of *Neurology* indicated that Alzheimer's patients who took nonsteroidal anti-inflammatory drugs had better scores on 14 of 15 different cognitive tests and experienced smaller declines on test scores over the course of a year than did Alzheimer's patients who did not take the drugs. A large clinical trial is currently under way to determine if **prednisone**, a steroid, can slow the course of Alzheimer's.

Q: I guess there are no drugs being studied that could actually prevent or cure Alzheimer's, are there?

A: Not yet. As researchers become more knowledgeable about the causes of Alzheimer's, however, they will be better equipped to develop treatments to prevent or cure the disease. If, for example, they determine that beta amyloid does play a role in neuron death, they can turn their attention to drugs that stop it from accumulating or that inactivate it. If they find that tau is a factor, they will look for drugs to prevent the protein from developing into tangles. If they learn more about the roles of the different variants of ApoE, they may develop drugs to either mimic the protective effects of ApoE 2 or stop the destructive effects of ApoE 4. For now, however, drug research is focusing primarily on drugs that slow the progress of the disease or improve the symptoms.

TREATMENTS FOR DEMENTIA SYMPTOMS

Q: Did you say there are medical treatments for some dementia symptoms?

A: Yes. Both medical treatments and nonmedical techniques can be used to manage certain dementia symptoms, including anxiety, agitation, sleep disturbances and depression. In some instances, medical treatments are preferable; in others, nonmedical techniques are preferable; and in still others, a combination of both works best.

Q: I can see why a combination of the two might work best, but why would nonmedical techniques be preferable to medications in some instances?

A: Because some medications can cause adverse reactions or side effects or interact with other drugs a person is taking. Remember, adverse drug reactions and interactions are a common cause of dementia symptoms. They can also exacerbate dementia symptoms in people who have a dementing illness. As

you recall, the body's method of breaking down drugs changes
with age, altering appropriate doses for elderly individuals. And
the majority of people with dementia are over 65. Because of
this, medications are not always the best ways for dealing with
dementia symptoms.

Q: Are there any precautions that can be taken to
make the drugs safer?

A: Yes. For starters, any drugs prescribed to a person with
dementia should be prescribed in the smallest dose that
proves to be effective. This can help avoid overdosage and adverse
drug reactions. In addition, someone should maintain a list of all
the drugs the person is taking, and every doctor involved in treating that person should be notified of all the drugs he is taking.
This can help avoid and identify adverse drug interactions. Finally,
the caregiver should make sure her charge is taking all drugs
exactly as directed and keep a record of any side effects or problems that occur. If problems do occur, they should be reported
to the doctor immediately.

Q: Okay, I've been warned. Which dementia symptoms
can be treated with medications?

A: The symptoms and behaviors that can be treated or controlled to some extent with medications include agitation
(including wandering and violence), anxiety, hallucinations, delusions, paranoia, depression and sleep disturbances.

Agitation and Anxiety

Q: What types of drugs are used to treat or control
agitation and anxiety?

A: Three major types of drugs are used to treat agitation and
anxiety and their resulting behavioral problems, such as
wandering and violent behavior. They are antipsychotic drugs,
antianxiety medications and antidepressants.

Q: Could you tell me more about antipsychotic drugs?

A: Certainly. Antipsychotic drugs, also known as **neuro-leptics** or major tranquilizers, include:

- phenothiazines, such as chlorpromazine (Thorazine), thioridazine (Mellaril) and fluphenazine (Permitil, Prolixin)
- haloperidol (Haldol)
- thiothixene (Navane)
- molindone (Moban)

Some of these names may sound familiar to you. We discussed some of them in Chapter 2 when we discussed drugs that can cause adverse reactions and produce symptoms similar to dementia. For this reason, it is important that these drugs be used with caution in treating people with dementia. Although they can have a tranquilizing effect and normalize mood, thought and behavior, they can produce such side effects as the following: drowsiness, low blood pressure, blurred vision, dry mouth, constipation, and Parkinson-like reactions such as trembling, stiffness and a masklike facial expression. Less common, but more serious, adverse effects include such dementia symptoms as agitation, insomnia, depression and disorientation.

Q: What about antianxiety drugs? Do they have the same problems?

A: Antianxiety medications, also known as minor tranquilizers, consist primarily of:

- benzodiazepines, such as diazepam (Valium), flurazepam (Dalmane), alprazolam (Xanax), temazepam (Restoril), chlordiazepoxide (Librium) and lorazepam (Ativan)
- buspirone (Buspar)
- propranolol, a beta blocker that, while not officially approved for use as an antianxiety medication, is often used for that purpose

Benzodiazepines may effectively reduce anxiety and agitation, but they take a while to break down and can build up in the body over time. These drugs can also produce certain side effects,

such as drowsiness, lethargy and unsteadiness, and other adverse
effects, such as dizziness, blurred vision, slurred speech, excite-
ment, agitation, anger, hallucinations, confusion, depression
and irritability.

Q: What about antidepressants?

A: The types of antidepressants most commonly prescribed
for people with dementia are tricyclic antidepressants,
such as amitriptyline (Elavil, Endep) and nortriptyline (Aventyl,
Pamelor), and monoamine oxidase inhibitors, such as phenelzine
(Nardil).

Antidepressants produce side effects—drowsiness, dry mouth
and blurred vision, for example. They can also produce other
adverse effects, including an unsteady gait, tremors, confusion,
hallucinations, agitation, restlessness, impaired memory and
Parkinson-like reactions.

Q: I can see why medication is not always appropriate
for people with dementia. Did you say there are
other ways to deal with these symptoms and
behaviors?

A: Yes. And we discuss the nonmedical techniques for dealing with dementia symptoms and behaviors in Chapter 7.

Hallucinations, Delusions and Paranoia

Q: Good. In the meantime, what type of drugs can
be used to treat hallucinations, delusions and
paranoia?

A: Primarily antipsychotic drugs like those we discussed
above. These drugs can be quite effective at controlling
these symptoms, but as we've indicated, they can produce
side effects.

Depression

Q: I assume depression is treated with antidepressants?

A: Yes. Retrospective reviews and case studies suggest that medical management can improve depressive symptoms in between 35 and 85 percent of people with dementia, although no studies have shown one antidepressant to be better than another in people with both depression and dementia (*Internal Medicine News,* October 15, 1995).

In early stages of dementia, psychotherapy, or "talk therapy," can also be helpful, and **electroconvulsive therapy**—a treatment in which a low-voltage current is sent to the brain through electrodes placed either on both sides or on one side of the scalp to induce a generalized seizure or convulsion—is also used to treat depression in people with mild dementia. Although these therapies become less effective as cognitive and language abilities decline, modified psychotherapy, music therapy and art therapy may provide some benefit in later stages. We discuss the importance of music, art and other activities in people with dementia in more detail in Chapter 7.

Sleep Disturbances

Q: What about sleep disturbances? How are they treated?

A: Sleep disturbances are generally treated with sedative hypnotic drugs—generally benzodiazepines, such as diazepam (Valium), flurazepam (Dalmane), temazepam (Restoril), chloral hydrate (Noctec), glutethimide (Doriden), ethchlorvynol (Placidyl) and triazolam (Halcion).

As you may recall, benzodiazepines also function as antianxiety medications, or minor tranquilizers. They are effective, but their side effects and adverse effects, listed above, are undesirable in people with dementia.

Q: It sounds like these drugs all work, but there are so many possible problems associated with them. Is it worth trying them at all?

A: That depends on the seriousness of the symptoms and behaviors being treated, the effectiveness of nonmedical techniques and a person's individual reaction to the various drugs. For one thing, not all people with dementia will experience side effects and adverse reactions from the drugs used to treat dementia symptoms. And even when side effects do occur, in some cases they are less dangerous than leaving the symptom or behavior untreated. Then again, many people with dementia respond well to nonmedical management techniques and do not need drug therapy at all. And others benefit from a combination of the two.

To sum it all up, medical treatment of dementia symptoms is a highly individual matter—one that should be based on the interest of the patient, not simply of the family, and on the advice of a doctor who is aware of the possible consequences and is willing to search for alternative solutions if necessary.

Q: What kind of alternative solutions are you referring to?

A: Either alternative drugs or the nonmedical management techniques we discuss in Chapter 7.

6 LIVING WITH DEMENTIA: AN OVERVIEW

Q: I know you said it's possible to improve the quality of life for people with dementia, and I know medical treatments can help, but it all sounds so hopeless. How can a person with dementia or a caregiver cope?

A: There is only one way: by learning to live with dementia. This is by no means an easy task. Dementia is an illness with wide-reaching consequences: It robs a person of his memory, abilities, independence and personality, and it robs a family of one of its members in a particularly heart-wrenching way. Living with dementia is difficult for the person himself, who must give up his independence and live in a world that is becoming increasingly complex, foreign and frightening. It is also difficult for the family caregivers, who, in addition to watching their loved one's mental acuity and health decline, must accept changes in their family roles and changes in their own lifestyles as they assume increasing responsibilities—both for their loved one's daily care and for any family responsibilities he held before becoming ill.

Q: That could include earning money, couldn't it?

A: Yes. If the person was the family's primary breadwinner, another family member may have to find a job. Even if his earnings contributed only part of the family income, the family may still have to find a way to make up for this loss. And dementia care itself is not without cost. Alzheimer's disease alone costs the nation approximately $100 billion a year, according to the Alzheimer's Association. That figure includes the cost of home care, medical care and nursing-home care. If family caregivers were paid for their efforts, the average annual cost of home care for a person with dementia could reach $47,000. And only about $12,000 of that is covered by insurance on average. Since those who provide care in nursing homes do receive payment for their work, nursing-home care is even more expensive. The average cost of nursing-home care is $36,000 per year per person, but the cost varies regionally and can exceed $70,000 in some areas.

Despite these overwhelming obstacles, people with dementia and their families find ways to cope. They do it by learning as much as they can about the illness causing dementia, anticipating and preparing for future needs and taking one day at a time. Quite simply, they cope by developing a plan to live with dementia. It can be done.

Q: **But it's such an overwhelming task! When does it start?**

A: It starts the moment someone realizes something is wrong. This could be long before a diagnosis is made— when the person experiencing symptoms first realizes that there is a problem and begins to compensate for her deficiencies, perhaps by making lists or avoiding complex social situations. Or it could be when a family member first recognizes a change in a loved one and sets up a doctor's appointment. But whenever the process starts, it should begin in earnest once a diagnosis has been made.

Q: **What is the first step of this process?**

A: The first step is to learn as much about the underlying illness as possible: which symptoms are possible; when those symptoms might appear; how the disease will progress; what treatments, if any, are available; what complications might develop; and what assistance will be needed in both the short- and long-term. This knowledge can help everyone involved— including the person with dementia—gain an understanding of that person's needs.

THE NEEDS OF PEOPLE WITH DEMENTIA

Q: I know needs are individual, but do people with dementia have any general needs I should know about?

A: They certainly do. To begin with, a person with dementia needs medical care. This is important not only for people whose conditions or symptoms can be medically treated, but for all dementia patients. Like everyone else, dementia patients can suffer from colds, flu, infections and other common ailments, as well as complications of their underlying illness. But many people with dementia are unable to recognize the symptoms of these ailments or communicate their needs. A knowledgeable physician knows what to look for and can teach caregivers how to prevent certain complications of dementia.

Q: What type of doctor provides medical care for people with dementia?

A: A number of doctors are capable of caring for dementia patients. Family practitioners, or general practitioners—doctors trained to prevent, diagnose and treat a wide variety of ailments in patients of all ages—can provide dementia patients with the routine care they need. So can internists—doctors trained in internal medicine.

With additional training, both family practitioners and internists can specialize in geriatric medicine—the care and treatment of the elderly. **Geriatricians** are usually well versed in the dementing illnesses common to the elderly as well as other diseases and conditions of aging. Geriatricians and neurologists—doctors who specialize in diagnosing and treating diseases and impairments of the brain and nervous system—are the specialists who care for dementia patients.

Q: Which doctor is best?

A: That depends on the person's specific needs. For routine care, a family practitioner, general practitioner or internist is fine. If the person has a number of other chronic problems related to his age, a geriatrician may be a better choice. And if the person wants to participate in research to help experts gain a better understanding of his illness or the effectiveness of experimental drug treatments, his best bet is to contact a neurologist.

Q: Why would a person want to participate in research?

A: Remember, doctors are not yet sure what causes Alzheimer's disease. And while they know what causes some of the other diseases that bring on progressive dementia, they have not found effective treatments or cures. A person with Alzheimer's disease or another dementing illness might have an altruistic desire to do something to further the understanding of her disease, or she might wish to participate in trials of experimental drugs in the hope that the drugs will improve her condition. As we indicated in Chapter 5, a number of treatments for Alzheimer's disease are being studied. The only way researchers can find out if these drugs effectively alleviate the symptoms or slow the progression of Alzheimer's disease is to give them to people who have the disease. The same holds true for treatments of other diseases as well. For more information about participating in research, contact the Alzheimer's Association, listed in the Informational and Mutual-Aid Groups section at the back of this book.

Q: What other general needs do dementia patients have?

A: As their mental abilities decline, dementia patients may need help making decisions and planning for the future. This can include short-term decisions, such as how to pay the bills or what to wear on a given day, and long-range decisions about end-of-life medical care and estate plans. As abilities deteriorate further, dementia patients require more and more supervision to keep them from causing harm to themselves and others and, eventually, assistance with daily activities, such as dressing, bathing, eating and toileting. And throughout the entire course of their illness, dementia patients need emotional support and understanding.

MEETING NEEDS

Q: **Those needs sound pretty daunting in an adult— particularly the supervision and help with daily activities. How can they be met?**

A: The need for supervision and help with daily activities is indeed unusual in an adult. A person with dementia must be constantly watched to make sure he doesn't leave the stove on, scald himself in the shower or wander—or drive—off and get lost. If the person with dementia is being cared for at home, family members must make efforts to make the home safe, put locks on the doors and take away the car keys or even remove the distributor cap from the car to prevent him from driving it. They must also learn how to help their loved one get dressed, eat and bathe. In Chapter 7, we discuss methods to make a home safe and help a person with daily activities.

Q: **Is family home care the only option for meeting the needs of a person with dementia?**

A: No. There are many ways to meet those needs: home care provided entirely by a family; family home care supplemented with help from friends, neighbors and community organizations; family home care supplemented with homemaking help; family home care supplemented with the services of a **home health agency**; family home care supplemented with **adult day care**; and differing levels of nursing-home care.

Q: Slow down a minute. I understand how friends, neighbors and community organizations might be able to help, and I can see the value of homemaking help. But what kind of services can a home health agency provide?

A: Home health agencies, which we discuss in detail in Chapter 7, can provide nursing services, homemaking services, supervision and help with daily activities.

Q: And adult day care?

A: Adult day care, like day care for children, provides organized programs of activities outside the home for adults who need supervision. Adult day care provides the family caregiver with a needed break and the adult being cared for with an opportunity to socialize with others. We discuss this in more detail in the next chapter.

Q: What about nursing-home care? Will we discuss that later as well?

A: Yes. Nursing-home care is discussed in detail in Chapter 8.

Q: Which of these caregiving options is most common?

A: That's hard to say. Many families of dementia patients— more than 70 percent, according to the Alzheimer's Association—choose to care for their loved ones at home, for at least part of the illness. Some supplement that care with adult day care, the services of a home health agency, help from friends, neighbors and community organizations or some combination thereof. Other families, however, find that nursing-home placement is the best or only way they can meet their loved ones' needs. And many begin with some type of home care, then turn

to nursing-home care when they can no longer meet the growing
needs of their loved ones.

FORMULATING A PLAN

Q: How do families decide what's best for them?

A: By sitting down together to outline the patient's current
and future needs and developing a plan that will meet
those needs as well as the needs of others in the family.

Q: That doesn't sound like an easy task!
Can't disagreements arise?

A: They certainly can. In fact, disagreements are common.
For one thing, different family members may view the
situation in different ways: Family members who live at a distance
or do not have regular contact with the patient may deny that
dementia exists, while those who are in close contact may see the
full extent of the problem and know firsthand that help is needed.
In addition, some family members may be more willing or better
able to help out than others, and disagreements may arise over
which member should assume which responsibility. Even if these
disagreements never materialize, family members may simply have
different opinions about what is best for their loved one.

Q: What if the family agrees on and implements a
plan but later realizes that it doesn't meet their
loved one's needs?

A: They simply return to the planning process. Initial planning is only one part of the process of learning to live
with dementia. Trial and error are common, especially since the
needs of both the patient and her family members may change
many times throughout the course of the illness. Remember, the
plan is designed to meet the needs of both the patient and the
family. When those needs change, so should the plan.

Q: What are some of the issues families should consider before formulating their original plans?

A: Individual family situations dictate some of those issues, but there are other issues all families must address before they decide how they can best meet their loved one's needs. Among the questions they must raise are:

- What type of care does the person need now?
- What type of care will the person need in the future?
- What types of care (nursing-home care, adult day care, home health care and so forth) are available in the area?
- What do the various types of care cost?
- What financial resources does the person have?
- Is the person eligible for any financial assistance?
- Are any family members willing or able to pay for care if the person cannot?
- What roles can various family members play in caring for their loved one?
- If care is to take place in the home, is someone willing and able to assume the role of primary caregiver?
- In whose home would home care take place?
- Is that home located near family members and necessary services?
- What must be done to make that home safe for the person with dementia?
- What type of arrangements can be made to care for the person if the caregiver becomes ill?

Q: Couldn't the person with dementia answer some of those questions himself?

A: Depending on the person's abilities, he can be of great help in developing a plan for his own care. He may have definite opinions about where he wants to live, what type of care he wants and doesn't want, and how his financial matters and estate should be handled. This is one of the greatest advantages of early diagnosis—the patient may be able to actively participate in plans for his future.

PLANNING FOR THE FUTURE

Q: Let's say the person's mental capabilities are still relatively intact. What type of long-term plans should he help make?

A: If he knows and accepts the fact that his disease will eventually render him incapable of making important decisions and, ultimately, lead to his death, he will probably want to make out his will, get his insurance policies in order and decide on key issues relating to his health care. He may also want to assign a family member or friend to make decisions for him when he is no longer able.

Financial Planning

Q: You mentioned a will and insurance policies. Could we discuss these and other financial considerations in a little more detail?

A: Yes. Let's start with the will. The person needs to prepare a will if he hasn't already.

Q: Can someone with dementia prepare a valid will?

A: That depends upon his mental condition. Specific laws regarding this may differ from state to state. But according to *Caring for the Alzheimer Patient: A Practical Guide,* as long as the person still knows the nature and extent of his property, is still able to formulate a distribution plan and understands the relationship between himself and those to whom he's leaving property, his will should be valid.

Q: Is there anything else I should know about wills?

A: Yes. It's one thing to have a valid will; it's another thing to know where to find it when it is needed. The person needs to inform family members where his will is kept and provide them with the name of his lawyer. The same holds true for other important documents and consultants. For example, someone should know where insurance policies, bank accounts, stock certificates and other documents are kept, as well as the names of the patient's accountant, stockbroker and the banks with which he deals.

Q: That makes sense. But what if the patient is further along in his illness and can't provide that information?

A: Then family members or friends have to do some investigating. They might be able to find some of the information they need—account numbers, property holding and outstanding loans, for example—on old bills, bank statements, canceled checks and tax forms. Other information might be more difficult to find, however.

Q: What other long-term financial issues might the person want to address?

A: Primarily matters that can assure that his care will be paid for and that his loved ones will be financially secure after his death. If he receives a pension or other retirement benefits, for example, he might want to refresh himself about the plan's provisions for paying benefits after his death and double-check that the beneficiary he has named is still the person he wishes to receive the money. Or he might wish to make arrangements to have the pension check sent to someone else if he becomes incompetent.

Likewise, he might want to make sure that any insurance policies he has are up to date and make provisions to keep them that way—i.e., arrangements to have premiums paid after he is no longer able to do so. He might want to look once more at whom he has named as beneficiary of his life-insurance policy or check with his health-insurance agent to determine if any of the care he will need during the course of his illness will be covered. And he might want to investigate purchasing a long-term-care policy to cover his future health-care needs.

Q: It almost sounds like you're saying the person with dementia must prepare for death! Are you?

A: In a sense. Although he may live for years with his condition, in the final stages he may not be able to make the important decisions he needs to make before death. If he wants to have a say in those matters, he needs to do it early.

Q: I understand. But in the same vein, he may not be able to handle his day-to-day financial decisions either. Is there any way to assure that these decisions can be made once the patient becomes unable to do so?

A: There are several possible solutions to this problem, all of which involve the legal delegation of decision-making authority. The most common methods used by someone who has not yet lost his ability to make decisions are **power of attorney** and **trusts**. Both of these methods enable the patient to assign a person or persons to act on his behalf.

Q: What is the difference between the two?

A: Power of attorney permits a second individual to make decisions for another person as if that person had made the decision himself. Someone who has power of attorney can write checks, pay bills and make other financial decisions for another person. She can also make other legal decisions—for example, entering into a contract or deciding on nursing-home placement. Essentially, she is able to act as if she were the person she is representing.

Trusts, on the other hand, are primarily financial. They allow one or more persons or institutions (such as a bank) to be named to *manage* the property, assets and other financial matters of a person. They, too, enable someone else to pay bills and make financial decisions, but in this case that individual acts as a trustee over specific assets deposited in the trust, not as the owner's representative.

Q: Which is better?

A: That depends on the goals and needs of the person and his family. An attorney who specializes in estate planning can advise the person with dementia and/or his family as to whether either or both are appropriate in a particular situation.

Q: Both of those methods require the person to designate his own representative. Can either be established if the person no longer recognizes anyone around him?

A: Yes, but not by the person himself. If the person has already lost the ability to make such a decision, a legal proceeding must be sought to grant decision-making power to others. After the court is petitioned, hearings are held to determine the patient's limitations and needs. If it is determined that the person is no longer capable of handling his own affairs, the court will grant power of attorney to someone—usually a family member or friend—or appoint someone to act as that person's **guardian**. In guardianship, the court gives the guardian the responsibility of caring for that person and the authority to manage his affairs.

Health-Care Planning

Q: Are there similar legal provisions to handle health-care decisions?

A: There are. Health-care decisions can be made by means of **advance directives**—written documents that, in the case of a serious illness, either clarify an individual's wishes for health care or name a person to make health-care decisions for him if he becomes unable to do so. The two most common types are **living wills** and **durable powers of attorney for health care**.

Q. They sound similar to the estate provisions.
Are they?

A. Yes. A living will, like a regular will, enables a person to outline specific wishes. In the case of a living will, those wishes are specific to health care. A living will describes what types of medical treatments a person will permit in order to prolong her life: for example, whether or not she wishes to be put on a respirator and in what instances, and whether or not she wants to be fed via tube or IV when she can no longer feed herself.

A durable power of attorney for health care, like the power of attorney described earlier, enables a person to designate another person to make decisions for her—in this case, decisions about health care. The document transfers health-care decision-making power to a designated representative in the event that she becomes unable to make her own health-care decisions. It can also specify what treatments the person does or does not want to allow.

Q. Does a person with dementia need one or both?
Is one better than the other?

A. Again, that depends on the individual situation. The durable power of attorney for health care is quite different from a living will. It can be used to employ medical personnel, arrange for nursing-home care and consent to specific medical procedures, as well as to designate when life-sustaining treatment should or should not be used. Living wills are limited only to the latter. Many individuals elect to have both types of advance directive.

Q. How does one establish these advance directives?

A. The laws governing living wills and durable powers of attorney for health care differ from state to state, so it is best to consult a lawyer familiar with the laws of the state in which you live. Another source of help is Choice in Dying, which has a legal department that can provide further information on advance directives. For information on how to contact Choice in Dying, see the Informational and Mutual-Aid Groups section later in this book.

PUTTING THE PLAN INTO ACTION

Q: **Okay. Let's say the patient has taken care of these long-term issues and has helped the family develop a plan to meet his needs. What's next?**

A: Next, the family must put the plan into action. Remember, however, that the plan is not etched in stone. It can be changed at any time or at least adapted to fit the increasing or changing needs of the patient or family. Many families, for example, plan to care for their loved ones at home for the duration of their illnesses but then reach a point where they are physically or emotionally unable to do so. They then must change their plans. Some seek additional help, hiring helpers or enrolling their loved ones in adult day care; others find that nursing-home placement is the best option. Likewise, some families who initially turn to a nursing home for help later find out that they can provide more suitable care for their loved ones. Putting a plan into action is by no means the final step in learning to live with dementia.

Q: **How does a family go about putting their plan into action?**

A: That depends on the content of the plan. If the patient's daily care is to take place in a nursing home or other long-term-care facility, the family must choose a facility and make the appropriate arrangements. If care is to take place at home, the family must make sure the home is safe, and the primary caregiver must familiarize herself with what that care will entail. We discuss these caregiving options in the next two chapters.

7 HOME CARE

Q: Let's say my family decides to care for our loved one at home. Where should we start?

A: That depends on what your family has done before making that decision. Let's assume you've already learned something about your loved one's illness. Let's also assume that you've looked at the different housing options, financial issues and family concerns and have decided who will be the primary caregiver and where care will take place. At this point, your family should examine the home in question and do anything necessary to make it safe and secure. At the same time, the primary caregiver should learn as much as possible about the various techniques she can use to help with daily care. And, if your family hasn't already done so, it should investigate the services available in the area that may be helpful in the future.

PREPARING THE HOME

Q: Let's start with the home. What do you mean— make it safe and secure?

A: Although your loved one may be no immediate danger to himself right now, that may change in the future. Remember, memory loss continues in progressive dementia; judgment can become impaired, and walking, balance and motor skills can decline. A person with dementia can accidentally harm himself with a sharp object, ingest something poisonous or trip and fall. And if he is a wanderer, he may leave the home when you are not looking, exposing himself to additional dangers. With this in mind, you need to "tour" the home early on and eliminate as many potential hazards as you can.

113

Q: It almost sounds as if you're talking about childproofing the home. Are you?

A: Although the situations are different, the concept is essentially the same. So, in fact, are many of the specific precautions to make a home safe. But because the person with dementia is an adult who is accustomed to performing many activities that, if done incorrectly, could be dangerous, additional precautions may be needed. For example, you may need to take steps to prevent a person with dementia from harming herself while she is cooking.

Q: I see what you mean. She could leave the stove turned on or cut herself. What exactly can we do to make our home safer for our loved one?

A: As we've just seen, some hazards vary according to the room in question; the kitchen and bathroom, for example, pose specific problems. But before we look at those, a number of things can be done in all rooms to which the person with dementia will have access. You can:

- Remove sharp, heavy or breakable objects and objects small enough to be put into a person's mouth, to prevent cuts, injuries, choking and other accidents.
- Install locks on all doors to the outside to prevent outdoor wandering.
- Insulate the hot surfaces of radiators and other heating devices to avoid burns.
- Tack down rugs or replace them with carpeting to avoid trips and falls.
- Tack down or move electrical cords to avoid trips and falls.
- Arrange furniture in a simple, uncluttered manner to allow for easy traffic flow.
- Install night lights to avoid nighttime confusion.
- Light all stairways and make sure they have railings.

Q: What additional precautions should be taken in the kitchen?

A: The major hazards in the kitchen are knives and other sharp objects, breakable items, household chemicals and appliances.

Knives and other sharp objects should be kept out of sight and out of reach. Breakable items and household chemicals should be moved or kept in cabinets with childproof doors and latches. The same goes for dangerous small appliances, such as electric knives and food processors. To make the stove safe, you can either remove stove knobs or install an out-of-sight, out-of-reach shutoff valve on gas stoves. Both of these options can prevent the stove from being turned on easily. Finally, access to the kitchen can be cut off entirely with the installation of a locked door, if necessary.

Q: There's no way you can lock a person out of the bathroom, but it poses as many dangers as the kitchen. What can we do to make it safer?

A: You can start by putting all poisonous substances, medications and sharp objects, such as razors and scissors, out of reach. Radios, hair dryers or other small appliances that could accidentally come into contact with water should also be placed out of reach or locked away. And you'll want to make sure the bathroom door can be unlocked from the outside as well as from the inside. (You don't want your loved one to lock himself in the bathroom unattended.)

To make the bathtub or shower safer, adjust the thermostat on your hot-water heater so that your loved one cannot accidentally scald himself, and place bath mats, decals or nonskid tape in the tub or shower to prevent slips and falls. You may also want to install grab bars or handles in the shower, or purchase a shower seat. This can make it easier for your loved one to get into and out of the tub; it can also make bathing easier when your loved one needs assistance.

Q: Are there any other things we can do to make our home safer?

A: Yes. Do whatever you can to make your home—your loved one's living environment—less confusing. Arrange furniture in simple, uncluttered ways, then leave it there; don't rearrange it. Make sure your house is well lit, and avoid unnecessary clutter.

Q: When you say unnecessary clutter, what do you mean? Should we remove all of our knickknacks?

A: No. In fact, it's important to keep familiar objects around. Familiar objects may help your loved one stay oriented. Pictures can prompt memories of people and events, and cherished personal belongings can help a person retain his sense of identity. Having too many items around, on the other hand, can cause confusion. You don't have to remove all your knickknacks, just reduce the number of them in rooms to which your loved one has access.

DAILY CARE

Q: Okay, we've taken care of the home. What else needs to be done?

A: At this point you're ready to start caring for your loved one. This involves not only meeting his physical needs and helping him maintain his health, but also working to assure his emotional well-being and coping with his behavior. Remember, this process can change from day to day. As your loved one's dementia progresses and his needs change, your responsibilities, activities and coping techniques will also change. Because of this, and because dementia progresses in different ways in different people, there are no set rules to guide you or surefire techniques for you to use. Several general guidelines may be of help, however, and numerous techniques are available to address the various problems that may arise. You simply have to find out which ones work best for you.

General Guidelines

Q: Let's start with the general, then move to the specific. What do I need to know about caring for a person with dementia?

A: Perhaps the most important thing to remember is to treat him with respect and help him maintain his dignity. While he may need the help and guidance you would normally give a child, he is an adult.

Q: But isn't it hard to keep that in mind when a person with dementia throws a temper tantrum or says something rude or tactless?

A: Yes. The troubling behaviors of people with dementia are hard to accept. They may seem like the willful behaviors of children testing the waters to see what they can get away with. But you must remember that these behaviors are the result of a disease that affects the ability to think clearly. They are not willful actions designed to annoy you, although they may indeed be deliberate.

Q: What do you mean, they may be deliberate?

A: In many cases, the troubling behaviors exhibited by people with dementia are legitimate expressions of need. Let's say a person with dementia is scared or frightened, for example. He may be unable to voice those emotions. In fact, he may not even recognize them, but he *can* react to them. The temper tantrum he may throw is a reaction to a legitimate fear. To give you another example, a person with dementia may feel hot, so he may take off his pants. He no longer understands that social conventions prohibit him from doing so in public; he simply feels the need to cool down and reacts accordingly.

With experience and a little investigation, you may be able to discover which specific problems have promoted troublesome behaviors. If you are successful, you may be able to end that behavior simply by correcting the problem. But even when you cannot pinpoint the specific cause of troublesome behavior, you need to remember that there is a general cause—dementia. In a person with dementia, actions are dictated by flawed thinking, not by a desire to be willfully annoying.

Q: That's good to know. What other general suggestions do you have about caring for a person with dementia?

A: Make sure she remains active and let her do as much as she possibly can. This will help her maintain her identity and a sense of purpose. It will also help her maintain her dignity. A person doesn't cease to exist the moment she has been diagnosed with dementia. She continues to live on—often for years. It is important to make those years as pleasant and meaningful as possible.

Q: I'm sure it is. But how do you determine what a person with dementia can and can't do?

A: By watching her. Some inabilities are obvious. Others are more subtle. She may, for example, suddenly stop doing something she likes to do or tell you she doesn't like it. She may forget the steps to a task—such as getting dressed—or perform the task incorrectly—perhaps putting her blouse on backward. Or she may express frustration. At that point, you may need to intervene—either by helping her or by doing it for her. While a person with dementia should be allowed and encouraged to do as much as she can by and for herself, she should not be forced into doing things she cannot do.

Q: That's understandable. Are there any ways a caregiver can help a person with dementia retain her ability to do things on her own?

A: Yes. In fact, that's one of the caregiver's primary tasks. Most caregivers find that establishing a routine—for daily activities and for life in general—can help the person with dementia stay focused and retain some of her abilities. Routines can help eliminate confusion. It's somewhat more difficult to forget to eat breakfast, for example, if you eat it at the same time every day.

In addition to establishing a routine, the caregiver can look for ways to simplify activities or provide assistance in subtle ways. He can also look for things the person with dementia can do— especially meaningful things, such as housekeeping chores and recreational activities—and focus primarily on them.

Finally, the caregiver needs to remember to assign tasks or activities to a person with dementia one at a time. This can help avoid confusion on the part of the person with dementia. It also helps the caregiver cope. As we said in Chapter 6, caregivers are generally more successful if they take things one day—and one problem—at a time.

Activities of Daily Living

Q: As a caregiver, I assume I will face a number of tasks every day—tasks that should be included in the daily routine. Can you give me some idea what to expect?

A: Certainly. As a caregiver, one of your most important functions is to help your loved one perform what are considered **activities of daily living**. These activities, which include eating, drinking, dressing, bathing, grooming and toileting, are done by everyone nearly every day. At the beginning of your loved one's illness, he may not require any assistance with these activities, or he might simply need to be reminded to do them. As his illness progresses, however, he will require more and more assistance. And in the later stages, you may actually have to perform some of the activities for him yourself. Your goal as a caregiver is to see that these activities are performed and to make them as easy for your loved one as possible. Remember, you want him to do as much as he can for himself.

Eating and Drinking

Q: What are some of the things I can do to make eating easier?

A: Before we get into specifics, there are two general concepts you need to keep in mind. The first is that mealtime should be routine. We've already mentioned the importance of routine to a person with dementia, and the concept holds true for meals. Eat at a set time in a set place. Make mealtime pleasant, and don't rush.

The second is that meals should be nutritious. Your loved one needs certain nutrients to stay healthy. At some point in his illness, he may not remember what he should be eating or his tastes may change; he may lose his appetite altogether; or he may not remember that he's already eaten and be ready for a second meal minutes after finishing the first. Your job is to make sure that he eats and drinks what he needs to maintain his health and that he doesn't eat too much.

Q: Understood. What are some of the specific ways I can make eating easier?

A: During the earlier stages of dementia, you may want to:

- Limit the number of food choices available.
- Assist your loved one with his food selections.
- Serve one item at a time.
- Monitor the portions he takes or serve prepared portions.
- Cut food before serving it.
- Avoid serving excessively hot food.
- Provide plenty of napkins.
- Monitor fluid intake.
- Provide your loved one with plenty of time to eat.

As dementia progresses and eating skills diminish, you also may need to:

- Serve finger foods.
- Remind your loved one to chew.

- Serve soft, mashed or shredded food.
- Consider vitamin supplements, if necessary.
- Learn the Heimlich maneuver.

In the final stages of your loved one's illness, you may have to feed him yourself. And if he eventually becomes unable to swallow, he may need specialized feeding, via either IV or tube. If this occurs, you yourself might need help helping him.

Dressing

Q: **How about dressing? What can I do to make that easier?**

A: In the beginning, you may simply need to eliminate unnecessary accessories, such as jewelry, ties and scarves, and put signs or labels on your loved one's drawers or closets to remind him where his clothes are kept. Later you may need to limit his choice of clothing or lay out a specific outfit for him.

Q: **What kind of clothing should he wear?**

A: He should wear clothing that is both comfortable and easy to put on. Remember, dementia can affect motor skills. This can make buttons, shoelaces and other fasteners difficult to deal with. Step-in shoes, like loafers, and clothing with elastic waistbands or Velcro closures are easier to work with—both for your loved one and for you, when you must assist him in dressing.

Q: **How can I assist him with dressing?**

A: At first, by simply reminding him, step-by-step, what he needs to do to get dressed. You may, for example, need to hand him a pair of pants and tell him to put his left leg in the left pant hole. After he has done that, you may then need to tell him to put his right leg in the other pant hole. Next, you may need to tell him to pull up his pants, and finally, to fasten them.

Remember, dementia can affect the logical processes in the brain, including the ability to perform tasks with multiple steps. We simply think of getting dressed as getting dressed. We rarely stop to realize the number of steps it involves. A person with dementia may be physically able to get dressed even during the later stages of his illness, but he will need direction to do so.

Q: Even so, I assume at some point I'll have to dress my loved one myself. Am I right?

A: Yes. At first you simply may have to help him, perhaps by holding out an article of clothing—say, a shirt—and directing him to put his arms through the sleeves. Later, however, you may have to physically dress him yourself.

Bathing and Grooming

Q: Okay, we've helped him dress and we've helped him eat. How can we help him with his personal hygiene?

A: In the beginning, you may simply need to remind him that it's time for him to take a bath or shower, or that he needs to wash his hands, shave, or brush his teeth or hair. (An electric razor and a simple, easy-to-care-for hairstyle can be big helps here.)

Later, you may need to remind him how to do these things, by posting a list of step-by-step instructions in the bathroom, by labeling various items in the bathroom or by illustrating the various steps with pictures.

Eventually, however, you will have to be present with him in the bathroom to guide him through the various processes.

Q: What will I have to do?

A: Think for a minute about all of the steps involved in taking a shower or bath: You have to turn on the water;

adjust the temperature; take off your clothes (one piece and one body part at a time); step into the tub or shower; pick up the soap; wash yourself; rinse off; turn off the water; step out of the tub; pick up a towel; dry yourself off and get dressed (again, one piece of clothing and one body part at a time).

Imagine how overwhelming this process can be to a person with dementia. He may be physically capable of performing all those activities, but he may have great difficulty remembering the order in which he should do them.

Your role is to break the job down into individual tasks and give your loved one simple, direct instructions.

Q: Does the same hold true for other aspects of personal hygiene, like brushing teeth and combing hair?

A: It certainly does. You need to break the job down into individual tasks and tell your loved one exactly what to do.

Q: At some point, will I have to participate in a more hands-on way?

A: Yes. In the later stages of your loved one's illness, you may have to physically assist him with bathing, grooming and dental care. Eventually, you may have to perform these activities yourself. And if your loved one reaches the stage at which he loses his ability to control his muscles, bathing may, of necessity, consist of sponge baths, unless someone is available to help you get your loved one into and out of a bathtub.

Toileting

Q: Are there any other activities of daily living I can help with?

A: Yes. People with dementia may need help with toileting. This is, of course, one thing you can never actually do for someone. You may, however, need to remind him to urinate or defecate, remind him where the bathroom is and help him with the various activities—such as undressing, flushing, dressing and washing hands—that go along with the toileting.

Q: How exactly can I help?

A: For starters, you can put a sign on the bathroom door, identifying it as the bathroom. Later, you may find that signs reminding your loved one to wipe after urinating or defecating, to flush the toilet and to wash his hands are helpful. At some point, he may need reminders to go to urinate or defecate in the first place. And eventually, he may need to be accompanied into the bathroom and given step-by-step instructions on what to do.

Q: Didn't you say way back in Chapter 1 that people with dementia can become incontinent in the later stages of their illness?

A: We did. We discuss methods of dealing with incontinence in more detail later in this chapter. For now, however, you need to be aware that in the later stages of dementia, when a person becomes incontinent, your assistance in this particular activity of daily living may consist of dressing him in disposable undergarments, changing those undergarments, cleaning up after him and/or dealing with a urinary catheter.

Dementia Symptoms and Behaviors

Q: Now that I have some idea what daily care involves, tell me some of the things I can do to manage the specific problems or behaviors that may arise from day to day?

A: Gladly. Back in Chapter 5 we reviewed the medical treatments that can help alleviate some of the symptoms of dementia. In addition to those treatments, there are numerous nonmedical techniques caregivers can use to manage dementia symptoms and behavior and to improve the quality of life for people with dementia. And while the list may seem long and ex-

haustive, many of these techniques arise from the general guidelines we've discussed above—establishing routines; keeping your
loved one occupied; simplifying tasks; looking for the underlying
cause of problem behavior; and taking things one at a time. Keeping those basic ideas in mind may make these techniques easier
to remember.

Memory Loss

Q: That's good—there's already a lot to remember.
And speaking of memory, are there any techniques
I can use to help my loved one combat his
memory loss?

A: Yes, and we've already discussed a number of them.
For starters, it is important to minimize confusion to
help a person with dementia stay focused. This can be done by
establishing routines and eliminating distractions. Reminders—
either written or verbal—can also be a big help in combating
memory loss. In our discussion about activities of daily living, for
example, we suggested that you post a list of instructions in the
bathroom or provide verbal assistance, explanations and step-by-
step instructions.

Some caregivers also find it helpful to label rooms so their
loved ones can find their way around. Others find it helpful to
wait until immediately before something has to be done before
providing instructions. If there are many things for a person to
remember, a list might help. And physical cues, such as calendars
and clocks, can help him with time orientation.

Communication

Q: Next to memory loss, I think the communication
difficulties associated with dementia would prove
to be the most challenging for me handle. Are there
any ways I can make communication easier?

A: Yes. There are many things you can do to improve communication with a person with dementia. Remember,
however, that not all people with dementia experience the same

difficulties using or understanding language. The exact nature of the problem depends upon the illness that is causing dementia and the extent of brain damage the illness has caused. Techniques designed to alleviate some language problems will not work for others. There are, however, some general guidelines that can improve communication in many instances.

Q: **Could you list them for me?**

A: Certainly.

- Eliminate unnecessary distractions.
- Call the person by name.
- Get the person's attention before speaking.
- Make eye contact with the person when you are speaking.
- Speak in a low, pleasant tone.
- Use short words and simple sentences.
- Speak slowly and clearly.
- Give the person adequate time to respond.
- Repeat things if necessary.
- Find ways to rephrase what you've said if it hasn't been understood.
- Use emphasis and facial expressions to enhance your speech.
- Use gestures and body language if necessary.
- Provide written reinforcement or visual clues if necessary.
- Communicate one idea at a time.
- Don't abruptly change the subject.
- When giving directions, break them down by step and give one step at a time.
- Listen carefully.
- Don't speak for the person.
- Offer encouragement and praise.
- Remain calm and relaxed.

Q: I can see how those would be helpful. But how can I address specific language problems?

A: Let's follow our own advice and address each problem as it occurs. In the earliest stages of language dysfunction, a person with dementia might exhibit a delayed response between her words or sentences or lose track of what she was saying and begin to talk about something else. You can address the first problem by giving the person adequate time to say what she has to say and the second with simple reminders. You can, for example, ask the person a question to get her back on track.

Another problem she may experience is difficulty finding a certain word. She may talk around the word, using a description rather than using the word itself, or she may simply forget the word altogether. In the first instance, known as **circumlocution**, communication is unaffected. If she calls a pen "the thing you write with," she has succeeded in getting her message across. You needn't do anything other than indicate that you understand. In the second, you can ask questions to try to determine what she is referring to.

Q: How can I address some of the more serious language difficulties, such as the tendency to use incorrect words?

A: When a person begins to use words that are completely incorrect, listen closely to what is being said; you may be able to understand what is meant from context and supply the word yourself. If you cannot, you can ask questions or offer her specific words from which to choose. If you're discussing fruit, for example, you can ask her if she is referring to an apple or an orange. Descriptions and gestures can also be helpful.

Gestures, objects and questions can also be used later on, when the person is unable to supply entire thoughts, not simply isolated words.

Q: If I were having difficulty expressing entire thoughts, I'm not sure I'd want to talk at all. Do people who experience these difficulties ever withdraw from conversation?

A: They do. And this is not good. Withdrawal further isolates a person with dementia. It can also create a gap between the person and his caregiver. If your loved one stops talking, try to draw him out. Get his attention and ask him questions or show him objects—anything to provoke communication.

Q: I'm sure comprehension also presents difficulties for people with dementia. What type of problems might they have in understanding speech, and how can I help combat those problems?

A: Several comprehension problems are common. A person with dementia may, for example, ask you to repeat something over and over again. Perhaps she understood what you said, but forgot it before she was able to respond; perhaps she didn't understand in the first place. When it happens repeatedly—and it does—it can be very annoying. Be patient. Repeat yourself slowly, enunciating each word. If that doesn't work, try to rephrase the sentence, using other words. Or try writing the information down. Depending on the skills lost, a person may be better able to understand written language than verbal language. Or vice versa.

Q: Are there any other things I can do to make myself better understood?

A: Yes. If a person doesn't understand a word you are using, you can define it, explain it or point to it. If she doesn't understand concepts, you can use gestures, descriptions, illustrations, demonstrations and objects to communicate your point. You can also reinforce things you've said in writing or with pictures.

Q: What are some of the language problems that can occur in the final stages of dementia-related language dysfunction?

A: In severe stages, a person with dementia may babble, use nonsense words, repeat a word or phrase over and over again, or repeat what you have said; this is known as **echolalia**. There's not much you can do to stop this other than trying to distract him.

Q: What happens when the person's language skills are totally gone? Is there any way to communicate then?

A: That's when gestures, smiles, touch and a soothing tone take on even more meaning. Remember, they *are* ways of communicating.

Delusions and Hallucinations

Q: What should I do if my loved one suffers from delusions or hallucinations?

A: Delusions—believing things that aren't true—and hallucinations—seeing or hearing things that don't exist—are very real to a person with dementia, and they can be quite frightening. If your loved one experiences delusions—if, for example, he believes he's someone he's not—do not argue with him. On the other hand, do not encourage his mistaken notions of reality. Simply try to change the subject.

Hallucinations can present additional difficulties. If your loved one is seeing or hearing something that isn't there, he may be very frightened. In response, you need to be supportive and reassuring. Try to focus his attention on objects in the room or get him to move around. And look for possible triggers. As you may recall from our discussion of medication side effects, some medications can cause hallucinations.

Sleep Disturbances

Q: What about sleep disturbances? Are there any nonmedical ways to prevent a person with dementia from waking up in the middle of the night?

A: The problem is not that people with dementia wake up in the middle of the night. We all wake up in the middle of the night at one point or another. The difference is, we know it's still nighttime and go back to bed. A person with dementia may have lost all orientation to time, however. When he wakes in the middle of the night, he may think it is time to get up and start the day. This does not harm him, but it can put great strain on his caregiver and the established routine at home. There are, however, a variety of nonmedical techniques you can try to prevent your loved one from waking and becoming active in the middle of the night.

Q: What are some of those techniques?

A: For starters, make sure your routine schedule differentiates between night and day. Daytime activities should be active; nighttime activities relaxing. It is also important to set an amenable bedtime. If you put your loved one to bed at 7 P.M., he's likely to wake up before sunrise. People generally require six to eight hours of sleep.

Some other suggestions:

- Make sure your loved one's bed is comfortable.
- Limit daytime naps.
- Limit liquid intake shortly before bed.
- Make sure your loved one uses the bathroom before going to bed.
- Limit caffeine intake.
- Remain calm if your loved one wakes at night.
- Monitor his health carefully. Pain and illness can trigger sleep disturbances.
- If he tends to wander, make sure your doors are locked or that your home is equipped with an alarm system.

Wandering

Q: That reminds me. I've read about people with dementia who have wandered off and died of exposure or gotten hit by a car, and I'm afraid my loved one will wander out of my sight and into danger. Why do people with dementia wander?

A: Wandering is one of the most frustrating and dangerous behaviors associated with dementia. Often a sign that a person is feeling lost, frightened or lonely, it can also be prompted by a search for someone or something, a need to communicate or a desire to get away. In other instances, wandering might have a more specific cause. Let's say a man tries to leave the house every morning at 8 A.M.—the time he used to leave for work. In this case, his wandering is what is known as an **agenda behavior**— a behavior that has a goal and purpose. In this case, the purpose is to get to work. If the caregiver can recognize the agenda, she can take steps to meet that agenda and reduce wandering. In the example we just discussed, the caregiver might try to convince her loved one that he does not need to go to work or empathize with his desire to go to work, acknowledging an important aspect of his personality.

Q: Is there any way I can minimize the chances that my loved one will wander?

A: You can try the following:

- Increase his level of physical activity during the day.
- Distract him with activities when he appears restless.
- Surround him with familiar things to make him feel secure.
- Keep his environment free of disturbing sights and sounds that might upset him and make him want to go away.
- Make sure his physical needs are being met. (If, for example, he is hungry, he might wander in search of food.)
- Increase his contact with others.
- Make sure he knows he is not alone.

Q: Those techniques are fine as far as they go, but are there any things I can do to physically keep my loved one from leaving the house?

A: We've already discussed the importance of making sure doors can be locked. Installing an alarm system that sounds when doors are opened may also help, although it is a more expensive option. In extreme cases—if, for example, he continually heads for the nearest door and reacts violently when stopped—you may have to physically restrain him.

Q: What if he succeeds in leaving? Is there anything I can do to help assure his safety?

A: Yes. For starters, you can buy him some sort of identification—perhaps a bracelet or necklace—that lists his name, address, phone number and the fact that he is memory impaired. There are also electronic devices you can purchase that can monitor the whereabouts of the person wearing them. If you do discover that your loved one has gone, notify the police immediately and enlist others to help you search for him.

You may also consider participating in the Alzheimer Association's Safe Return Program.

Q: What is that?

A: It is an organized program that helps identify, locate and return memory-impaired individuals who get lost. The program provides an identity bracelet or necklace, clothing labels and wallet cards to identify the individual; registration in a national database; a 24-hour toll-free number to contact when an individual is lost or found; access to a national network of local law-enforcement agencies that can help find the missing person; and a national network of local Alzheimer's Association chapters to provide education, training and support to families and caregivers. For more information, call the Association at 800-272-3900.

Incontinence

Q: We talked briefly about incontinence when we discussed activities of daily living. I guess now is a good time to get back to the subject. Is incontinence always permanent?

A: That depends on what is causing it. If a health problem—an infection, diabetes or medication, for example—is responsible, treating that underlying problem may put an end to incontinence. If a memory problem is to blame, reminders might help. And if slow movement is at fault, bringing the person closer to the facilities or the facilities closer to the person might prevent future accidents. But when the person reaches the point at which he no longer has physical control of his bladder and bowels, incontinence can be permanent.

Q: Is there any way to tell whether incontinence is permanent?

A: Yes, but it may involve some investigation and a consultation with the doctor. You need to observe your loved one's bathroom habits. Ask yourself: When are accidents happening? How often? Is the problem regular or occasional? Does your loved one indicate that he's experiencing pain? Do accidents happen on the way to the bathroom? Did the problem start suddenly? The answers to these questions may help you determine the underlying problem. They may also help the doctor determine if a physical problem is responsible. Infections, diabetes, an enlarged prostate gland and medications can cause urinary incontinence, while infections, diarrhea and constipation can result in bowel incontinence. All of these conditions can be treated.

Q: What about the other causes of incontinence— memory problems and slow movement?

A: If the person simply forgets to go to the bathroom, scheduling regular, frequent bathroom visits or reminding her to go may eliminate the problem. If she moves too slowly to get to the bathroom and get on the toilet in time, you can rent a commode chair and place it close by. You can also make sure her clothing is easy to get on and off.

Q: And if incontinence is permanent?

A: Then you must deal with it. As we've said, disposable undergarments for adults are available. There are also products, such as disposable incontinence pads and rubberized sheets, to protect your bed, chairs and other furniture.

Anxiety and Agitation

Q: Do you have any suggestions for alleviating anxiety or agitation?

A: Not to sound like a stuck record, but here again, establishing a routine, avoiding confusion and keeping the person with dementia active can be quite helpful. And if the source of the anxiety or agitation can be determined, eliminating it may eliminate the problem altogether.

Q: What are some of the problems that prompt these reactions?

A: Some common causes are tiredness, hunger and boredom. These, obviously, can be addressed easily. If you suspect the person is tired, schedule a nap. If you suspect she is hungry, give her something to eat. If you suspect she is bored, offer additional activities or entertainment.

In any event, your own reaction to your loved one's behavior can have a profound effect. If you are calm and reassuring, you may be able to reduce your loved one's anxiety and agitation. If, on the other hand, you become agitated yourself, you may make the problem worse. The environment, too, can have an effect. Reducing levels of noise and confusion may reduce your loved one's levels of anxiety or agitation.

Catastrophic Reactions

Q: You just said that when a caregiver becomes agitated, she can make the problem worse. In what way?

A: When a person with dementia becomes highly agitated or angry, he may exhibit what is known as a **catastrophic reaction**. A catastrophic reaction is an emotionally violent response to a relatively insignificant incident. It can take the form of crying, outbursts of anger, verbal abuse or physical violence, such as striking, biting and punching.

Q: What touches off these responses?

A: They can be prompted by new or strange situations inside the home, by unfamiliar environments, people or noises, or by a change in routine. They can also be prompted by sheer frustration on the part of the person with dementia. If he doesn't understand what he has been asked to do; if he cannot make himself understood; if he is asked several questions at once or asked to perform a task that involves multiple steps; if he is being hurried; or if he is trying to do something he can no longer do, he may react violently.

Q: As a caregiver, how should I respond to a catastrophic reaction?

A: First and foremost, try to remain calm. Second, realize that the reaction is not a deliberate attempt to be nasty. The things your loved one may say and do may be hurtful and shocking, but he will soon forget them.

Q: That's good to know. But in the meantime, are there any things I can do to try to calm him down?

A: Yes. Move slowly, use unthreatening body language and talk to your loved one in a calm, soothing tone. Don't try to argue or reason with him. That may actually aggravate his behavior. If possible, try to distract him from the source of his irritation and reassure him that things will be all right.

Q: **What if his reaction places me in danger or my attempts to calm him down don't work?**

A: If violence is directed at you, protect yourself. Get out of your loved one's way or get behind a barrier of some sort. If your loved one does not calm down, you may need to physically restrain him. If you cannot do so, call police or emergency medical personnel.

Q: **Are there any ways I can prevent a catastrophic reaction from happening in the first place?**

A: You can minimize the chances that a catastrophic reaction will occur by sticking to your routine, simplifying tasks, taking things one at a time, finding jobs and activities your loved one can do, monitoring your loved one's health, offering him assistance when necessary, and refraining from rushing him or pushing him to do things he can no longer do. Bear in mind, however, that following this advice does not guarantee that your loved one will not react violently when agitated. It simply reduces the possible sources of agitation.

Other Problem Behaviors

Q: **What about other problem behaviors, such as obsessive behavior or rudeness? Do you have any general advice that can help with them?**

A: Yes. For starters, remember the general guidelines we discussed earlier in this chapter: Establish and maintain a routine, encourage the person to remain active, and look for what might be triggering the rude or obsessive behavior. You might find it helpful to keep a log of problem behaviors. The log may help you determine the underlying cause of the behavior.

In addition, you can try a standard behavior-modification technique—ignoring undesired or problem behaviors and rewarding desired behaviors. Let's say your loved one is continually making critical comments about you. Don't make a fuss. Just ignore them. If you get upset, it might provoke him into a catastrophic reaction. If, on the other hand, he remembers to put his dirty clothes in the laundry hamper or completes a task he is asked to do, reward him with praise, hugs, a special treat or a favorite activity.

Recreational Activities

Q: **You've mentioned activity throughout this discussion. It seems to be an effective technique for addressing a number of problem behaviors associated with dementia. What kinds of activities are appropriate for a person with dementia?**

A: That depends on the person and on her capabilities. In general, activities for people with dementia should be centered around their previous likes and tastes. People rarely lose interest in things they have enjoyed throughout their lives simply because they are experiencing declines in mental function. If their activities can be modified and simplified to meet their changing abilities, they can continue to enjoy things that caused them pleasure in the past and so retain an important aspect of their identities.

Q: **Could you give me an example?**

A: Certainly. Let's say a person has been a music lover all her life. In the early stages of dementia, she may be able to pursue that hobby as she always did, writing music or playing an instrument. But when these abilities disappear, she can still enjoy music. She can listen to recordings, sing familiar songs and even make music by clapping to the beat.

Q: **And a person who once enjoyed reading may later enjoy being read to. I think I see what you mean. Can you give me some examples of other activities that might be appropriate?**

A: Yes. In her book *Failure-Free Activities for the Alzheimer's Patient: A Guidebook for Caregivers*, Carmel Sheridan, M.A., suggests the following:

Exercise: walking, calisthenics and activity games, such as batting balloons, passing a ball, catching a beanbag or playing ring toss

Domestic activities: gardening, raking leaves, dusting, sweeping, mowing the lawn, mopping the floor, folding clothes or helping with food preparation

Crafts: making things like collages, scrapbooks and mobiles

Solo activities: reading, watching television, winding yarn, sorting things, lacing things or stringing things

Family games: bingo, charades, puzzles

Reminiscing: looking through a photo album, watching home movies and engaging in conversation

Other activities that many caregivers find successful are drawing, coloring, painting, working with clay, looking at picture books or children's books, telling stories and dancing.

Q: **What about activities outside the home?**

A: Those, too, can be important, particularly in the earlier stages of dementia, before the person becomes too overwhelmed by unfamiliar places, people and activities. Going out to eat, walking in the park, going to church and other outside activities may be enjoyed by the entire family.

OVERALL HEALTH

Q: Clearly daily care is more than just keeping a person active, addressing dementia symptoms and helping with activities of daily living. What health concerns should the caregiver be aware of?

A: As we said in Chapter 6, people with dementia are not immune to other illnesses. They are prone to the common ailments that affect everyone else, and they can experience physical complications from dementia as well. And if they are older, they may also have to put up with chronic conditions, such as arthritis and osteoporosis. With that in mind, it is important that people with dementia receive the medical care they need. The problem is they may not recognize their needs. That is where the caregiver comes in.

The caregiver needs to watch his charge for signs of illness, including an abrupt worsening of behavior, fever, flushing or paleness, a rapid pulse, vomiting or diarrhea, skin changes, refusal of food, headache, moaning, shouting, convulsions, swelling, respiratory problems and sudden incontinence. He also needs to check his charge for cuts, bruises and other injuries.

Q: Are injuries common?

A: They can be. Remember, dementia can affect a person's motor skills and balance. In addition, many people with dementia may suffer chronic conditions that can affect their motor skills. Because of this, falls—and their resulting injuries— are common among people with dementia.

Q: What can I do to prevent falls?

A: The primary action you can take is to minimize hazards. Think back to our suggestions for making the house safe: Make sure the rooms are well lit and uncluttered, install grab bars and railings, tuck in loose wires and extension cords, replace

throw rugs with carpeting and, if necessary, limit your loved one's
access to stairs. In addition, make sure your loved one has had his
vision checked, that he is wearing safe footwear and that he gets
enough exercise.

Q: What's so important about exercise?

A: Exercise is much more than an activity to keep your
loved one busy. It can also help him retain his motor skills
and balance, improve his circulation and help him sleep. In fact,
regular exercise is essential to your loved one's health.

Exercise, or at least movement, can help prevent **decubitus
ulcers**, also known as bedsores. Decubitus ulcers often develop
in people who are bed- or chair-ridden for long periods of time.
The lack of movement places continuous pressure on the skin
that covers bony areas, such as the hips and shoulders. This persistent pressure impedes blood flow and kills tissue. These sores,
which are treated by cleaning the area and applying topical medications, take a long time to heal and can be life-threatening if they
become infected.

Q: What if the person with dementia can no longer
exercise because of his physical or mental dis-
abilities? Is there anything a caregiver can do to
prevent bedsores?

A: Yes. If the person is still physically able to move—even
if he spends most of the day in a chair or bed—the caregiver can remind him to move at regular intervals. This temporarily relieves the pressure on his skin. If the person can no
longer move himself, the caregiver can periodically change his
position herself.

Q: That sounds like it's easier said than done. Is it?

A: It can be difficult, especially if the caregiver is smaller
than her charge. If this is the case, she may need to get

outside help or perhaps consider placing her loved one in a nursing home.

Q: Are there any other complications that can occur with dementia?

A: Yes. Dehydration, malnutrition, constipation, infection and pneumonia are among the most common. A caregiver can help prevent the first two by monitoring her charge's food and fluid intake. Food and fluid intake also plays a role in preventing constipation, although medication may be needed to treat it when it occurs. Infection and pneumonia, obviously, require a doctor's attention. But it is up to the caregiver to make sure that that attention is sought.

FINDING ASSISTANCE

Q: All this—from health care and leisure activities to behavior management and daily hygiene—seems to comprise a 24-hour day. And I have other responsibilities as well. Is there anywhere I can turn for help?

A: There certainly is. In fact, many services are available, from medical care to housekeeping services. These services, provided by home health agencies, private companies, service organizations, volunteers, friends and other family members, include medical care, nursing care, services of **home health aides** and **personal-care aides**, housekeeping, meal services and adult day care. And for the caregiver herself, there is **respite care**.

Q: Let's discuss these in order. What kind of medical services are available and from whom?

A: Depending on the patient's needs, both medical and nursing services can be provided in the home. Some doctors still make house calls, and visiting nurses are generally the keystone of most home health agencies. Both registered and practical nurses offer services in the home, including dressing wounds, changing catheters, monitoring vital signs and overall health status, administering medications, giving injections and monitoring special dietary regimens. They can provide round-the-clock services, if needed, or pay regularly scheduled visits.

Q: **How can I find home nursing care if I need it?**

A: Your family doctor may be able to recommend a home health agency that provides the nursing services you need. These agencies may be privately owned, hospital-based or, like the Visiting Nurse Associations of America, nonprofit in nature. But they all employ nurses who work solely in the patients' homes.

Home health agencies, which are usually listed in the yellow pages of the phone book under the heading "home health care," may also be able to put you in touch with home health aides and personal-care aides who can provide an assortment of helpful services.

Q: **What should I look for in choosing a home health agency?**

A: You want to find an agency that provides the specific services you need and an agency that provides quality care. Licensing requirements for home health agencies vary from state to state. If your state licenses these agencies, check with the state health department to find out if the agency you are considering has a current, valid license. If your state does not license home health agencies, find out if the agency is Medicare- or Medicaid-certified. Certification means not only that Medicare or Medicaid will cover services provided by the agency but also that the agency has met certain standards.

You should also determine if the facility is accredited. Two agencies—the Joint Commission on the Accreditation of Healthcare Organizations and the National League for Nursing—accredit home health agencies. (For more information, see the Informational and Mutual-Aid Groups section.) Accreditation, which is

voluntary, is like Medicare certification in that it indicates that
the agency has met certain standards.

Q: You said a home health agency can put me in touch
with home health aides and personal-care aides.
What exactly do they do?

A: Home health aides, usually supervised by a nurse, can
take vital signs, apply dressings and assist with activities
of daily living, such as dressing, bathing, toileting and feeding and
moving a chair- or bedridden patient to prevent decubitus ulcers.
Personal-care aides, or **home attendants**, primarily assist with
activities of daily living and help with housekeeping.

Q: How many hours of service do these aides provide?

A: That depends on the amount of help you need and are
willing to pay for.

Q: What if my loved one really doesn't need much
help—just some supervision and companionship?

A: Then you can hire a **paid companion** or a **sitter**, who
can stay with him in your absence or even while you
take care of other responsibilities in the home. These employees
can be hired for several hours or on a live-in basis. Some may
be willing to assume additional caregiving or housekeeping
responsibilities.

Q: You've mentioned a couple of helpers that provide
housekeeping services. Are there any other sources
of housekeeping help available?

A: Various housekeeping services—including cooking, shop-
ping, doing laundry and cleaning—are offered by nonprofit agencies and volunteer programs sponsored by churches

and other charitable organizations. Friends and other family members can also be tapped to help out. And, of course, for those willing to pay, there are private housekeeping services.

Q: Where can I find out about these services?

A: If your loved one is a senior citizen, your local agency on aging may be a good starting point. These federally funded agencies, which are usually listed in the phone book's blue pages, track services and finance programs for older people who live at home. The blue pages may also help you locate other service agencies in your area—including Meals on Wheels, senior-citizen centers and various other nonprofit and volunteer programs.

Q: Meals on Wheels? Isn't that just for shut-ins?

A: No. This national nonprofit agency, which operates numerous local branches with the help of volunteers, prepares and delivers meals for individuals who cannot prepare food themselves. This includes shut-ins, of course, but it also includes individuals who cannot prepare meals for themselves because of physical or financial problems.

Area senior-citizen centers are another source for prepared meals, although they generally require the recipient to go to the center to receive them.

Q: Are there any other sources for housekeeping services?

A: Certainly. A number of private housekeeping companies clean houses, prepare meals, shop and do laundry, although this is a more expensive route. Private laundry services also exist. Check your yellow pages to find the services available in your area. You might also consider hiring an independent housekeeper to provide whatever services you need. And don't overlook the services that other friends and family members can provide. Many friends and family members may want to help but not know what they can do. You have to tell them.

Q: What *can* friends and family members do to help?

A: The Alzheimer's Association has some excellent suggestions:

For starters, they can keep in touch by sending cards, calling or dropping in for a visit. They can also do little things, like supplying a meal, running an errand or surprising the caregiver with a special treat. They can learn what they can about the person's illness and how it affects the family; listen and talk to family members; provide support for the caregiver and all family members; plan activities to get the whole family out of the house; offer and do specific things to help out; and offer to stay with the person with dementia so the caregiver can have some time alone.

Q: Doesn't adult day care essentially do the same thing?

A: It can. Adult day care is much like child day care—it provides the participant with needed supervision and stimulating activities in a safe, comfortable setting during specified hours, usually during the workweek. This allows the caregiver to work, run errands or relax without worrying about leaving his loved one unsupervised.

Like child day care, adult day care requires the adult to be taken to the day-care site, where she will spend time with other adults. This helps alleviate isolation and provides her with opportunities to socialize.

Q: But sometimes people with dementia do not behave in socially appropriate ways. Do adult day-care programs welcome people with dementia?

A: Many do. In fact, some are designed specifically for people with dementia. And many caregivers find that their loved ones' behavior actually improves when they participate in a day-care program. The stimulation and socialization draw them out.

In later stages of dementia, however, when the person requires constant care and help with activities of daily living, day care ceases to be a valid option.

Q: I can see why. But it sounds like it would work for me now. Where can I find an adult day-care program?

A: Adult day care is becoming more common as the need for it increases. Programs can be found in community centers and churches, as well as in independent facilities set up specifically for that purpose. They can also be found in nursing homes. To find a program or center in your area, check the yellow pages of your phone book under day-care centers (adult) or the blue pages under services for the aging.

Q: What is respite care?

A: Respite care is care given to the person with dementia by someone other than the caregiver. Its purpose is to give the caregiver a respite, or break, from caregiving activities.

Q: What kind of options are available?

A: Scheduled visits from family and friends, as well as those of home health aides, personal-care aides, sitters and paid companions, can provide the primary caregiver with a needed break. So, too, can her loved one's participation in adult day care or a prescheduled, temporary stay in a long-term-care facility like a nursing home. Any situation that temporarily relieves the caregiver of the responsibility of caring for her loved one can serve as respite care.

Q: Even with all the help available, there may come a time when I can no longer handle the responsibilities of caregiving. What can I do then?

A: At that point, you will probably consider placing your loved one in a long-term-care facility. That is the topic of our next chapter.

8 WHEN HOME CARE IS INAPPROPRIATE

Q: At what point does the typical family decide to put their loved one in a long-term-care facility?

A: That depends on a number of factors, including the health and needs of their loved one and the health and needs of the caregiving family. If, for example, their loved one has reached the later stages of her illness and requires professional care around the clock, family members may no longer feel qualified or able to continue caring for her at home.

The decision may also be prompted by the physical and emotional health of the family caregivers. If the primary caregiver becomes physically ill or emotionally unable to continue caring for his loved one at home—if, for example, his stress level has reached a certain limit or other family members have reached limits of their own—the family may consider placing their loved one in a long-term-care facility. Generally speaking, however, most families try to keep their loved ones at home as long as possible.

Q: Why is that?

A: For one thing, long-term care is extremely expensive. The average cost of nursing-home care is $36,000 a year. And costs can reach up to $70,000 in certain areas of the country. For another, the decision to place a loved one in a nursing home or other long-term-care facility can be very difficult. Family members may disagree over whether their loved one should be placed in a nursing home at all. Some members may feel it is wrong; others may see it as necessary for the health or well-being of their loved one and themselves. Even when family members agree, the decision may prompt strong feelings of guilt and sadness. Many people feel that placing their loved one in a long-term-care facility is akin to abandoning her. An adult child, for example, may feel that he owes it to his parents to care for them until their deaths, since they cared for him throughout the course of his life. Likewise, a spouse who promised to remain with his partner in sickness and in health until parted by death may feel an obligation to literally fulfill that vow. And other family members may feel guilty about breaking promises they made to their loved one earlier in her illness. These natural reactions are complicated by the perception that nursing homes are places of isolation and loneliness where people go to die.

Q: **It certainly is a difficult decision for a family to make. Do families eventually come to grips with their decision?**

A: Yes. But it may take time. In addition to feeling guilty, family members may truly miss their loved one's presence in their home. Caregivers may experience a withdrawal from their caregiving responsibilities and be at a loss about what to do with themselves. And all family members may experience grief and mourning. These reactions can be strong—perhaps equal to or greater than the reactions they will experience upon the death of their loved one.

Q: **Why?**

A: Because nursing-home placement marks an end to their previous life with their loved one. They know she will never again live with them at home.

Q: **But long-term-care placement doesn't mean an end to family relationships, does it?**

A: No. In fact, relationships can continue and even improve once a family member has moved to a nursing home or other long-term-care facility. The move can relieve family caregivers of the physical burdens and responsibilities of caregiving, allowing them to devote more time to meeting their loved one's emotional needs. Instead of spending two hours helping their loved one bathe and dress, they can spend two hours talking with her. And family members can still play a major role in caring for their loved one, making sure she is surrounded by familiar objects, assuring she gets the care she needs and acting as her advocate when she cannot represent herself.

Q: You said family members have the ability to make sure their loved one gets the care she needs. How exactly can they do that?

A: By choosing a facility equipped to meet their loved one's needs and then monitoring the care she receives in that facility. If her care is substandard or inappropriate, it is the family's job to point out the various problems and move her to another facility if necessary.

Q: So the initial selection of a facility is extremely important. What kind of long-term-care facilities do families have to choose from?

A: Several types of long-term-care facilities are available. For individuals who need 24-hour nursing and medical care—those in the final stages of dementing illnesses—there are **skilled nursing facilities**, which offer nursing services similar to those given in a hospital. For those who need less care—those in earlier states of dementia—there are **intermediate care facilities**, which provide less-intensive care than skilled nursing facilities, and **residential care homes**, or **assisted living facilities**, which offer what is known as **custodial care** (room, board and personal services). Some long-term-care facilities offer all three types of care—in segregated sections within the facility but not usually within the same unit. And some offer care specifically designed for people with dementia.

Q: I didn't realize there are—at least theoretically—so many choices available. How can I determine which is most appropriate for my loved one?

A: Obviously, your choices are limited by what's available in your area. Further, the answer to your question depends in part on your loved one's physical needs. If he is able to function well on his own and needs only minimal assistance, a residential care home may be right for him. If he needs a lot of help with activities of daily living, is losing mobility or needs constant supervision, an intermediate care facility may be more appropriate. And if he has lost much of his mobility—if, for example, he is confined to a bed or requires assistance from someone else to walk—or he is unable to feed or bathe himself, is incontinent, can no longer communicate or has chronic conditions that require medical attention, he needs the services provided by a skilled nursing facility.

Q: What if he doesn't need those services now but may in the future? Can he move from one type of facility to another?

A: Yes. This is somewhat easier if the facility you've chosen offers different levels of care, but it is also possible for people to move from one facility to another.

Just bear in mind that adjusting to a new home and new routine may present problems for your loved one. If you expect his physical needs to change dramatically after he moves into a long-term-care facility, keep that in mind when you begin your initial search for an appropriate facility.

Q: Other than physical needs, what determines which type of facility is most appropriate?

A: Appropriateness is also determined by the programs and services a facility offers and, of course, the overall quality of care it provides. As we saw in Chapter 7, people with dementia respond well to some forms of caregiving and poorly to others. Facilities in which staff members issue orders but don't offer explanations, offer few or inappropriate activities or use medications and restraints to control behavior will not meet the needs of people with dementia. Those that provide residents with individual attention, offer plenty of diverse activities and look for individual ways to control behavior, on the other hand, can enhance their residents' quality of life. We'll talk about the types of programs and services you should look for in a moment, but first we need to address quality of care.

Q: I guess you're right. I certainly don't want to put my loved one in a facility that has an excellent activity program but doesn't meet his basic physical needs. How can I make sure I'm dealing with a quality facility?

A: For starters, make sure it is licensed. Licensing, which is usually done by the state—either a dedicated board of nursing-home licensing or a facilities-licensing division within the department of health—assures that the facility meets minimum standards in areas such as fire and safety, housekeeping, maintenance, standards of care and staffing. In fact, facilities cannot operate legally without a license.

Q: Then what's the point of making sure they have one?

A: While it is true that licensing tells you little about the actual quality of a facility, it does tell you whether or not you're dealing with a legitimate operation.

Q: Okay. But obviously I need more to go on to determine whether a facility offers quality care. What else can I look for?

A: You can also look for a facility that has been Medicare- and Medicaid-certified. This indicates not only that Medicare and Medicaid will pay for covered services provided by that facility, but also that the facility has met certain standards.

Q: That reminds me. Will Medicare or Medicaid pay for long-term care?

A: Medicare does not cover what we generally think of as nursing-home care. It pays only for care in skilled nursing facilities for a limited time after hospitalization (up to 100 days a calendar year) and generally only for rehabilitative care.

Medicaid pays for traditional nursing-home care, but only for people with limited incomes and assets. Check with your local welfare office to determine whether or not you are eligible.

Q: Okay. Getting back to the quality issue, I should look for a facility that is licensed and Medicare- and Medicaid-certified. Anything else?

A: Yes. Some facilities also go through an accreditation process. Accreditation is voluntary and, like Medicare certification, indicates that the facility has met certain standards. The Joint Commission on the Accreditation of Healthcare Organizations is the agency that accredits long-term-care facilities. For information on how to contact the commission, see the Informational and Mutual-Aid Groups section at the back of this book.

Q: Do licensing, certification and accreditation guarantee high quality?

A: Not necessarily. They guarantee only that a facility has met certain standards. To really determine whether a facility offers the quality you are looking for, you need to tour it and ask specific questions.

Q: How do I arrange that?

A: What you must now do is call the facility or facilities under consideration for appointments. Make it clear that you not only want to talk to the facility's administrator, but you also plan to make an extensive tour. This will undoubtedly take an hour or more, so plan accordingly.

Q: What should I look for during my tour?

A: Look for:

Safety features: well-marked exits; smoke alarms; well-maintained sidewalks; fire extinguishers and/or a sprinkler system; ramps, handrails; grab bars on the toilets and bathtubs; nonslip surfaces in the bathtubs; locks, alarms or other provisions to prevent wandering

Overall livability: neat, well-maintained buildings; wheelchair ramps; wide, uncluttered corridors; spacious, well-maintained grounds; clean lobby; no unpleasant odors

Rooms: clean, spacious rooms; adequate closet and dresser space; nice furnishings; air conditioning; individual room thermostats; proximity to bathroom; adequate personal space; windows

Personnel: licensed, certified and qualified personnel (R.N.'s, physical therapist, occupational therapist, speech pathologist, dietitian, nurse practitioner); a physician on the premises a fixed time each day or, if not, available on call 24 hours a day; adequate number of aides (high ratio of aides to residents); pleasant demeanor; respectful treatment of residents

Recreational and social arrangements: numerous, varied activities; adequate personnel to plan and implement activities; a generous visiting policy; frequent outings for residents who are able to participate

Food: clean kitchen; clean dining area; varied menu; appetizing food; accommodating meal schedule; ability to accommodate special dietary needs; help available for eating

Q: Back up a bit. How easy is it to judge a facility's staff based on a brief tour?

A: You've asked a very good question. No matter how impressive the physical layout of a building, no matter how beautiful the grounds or how cheerful and spacious the rooms, no facility can be a decent place to live or deliver high-quality care if its staff is not qualified, dedicated and well-supervised.

Just remember the three basic features to look for: the availability of key personnel, their qualifications and their demeanor toward the residents.

Q: **Will every facility employ a variety of staff professionals?**

A: No. Although many facilities may not be large enough to have an occupational therapist or a speech pathologist on staff 100 percent of the time, all should have easy access to these professionals when the need arises.

Q: **What else should I find out about?**

A: You need to ask:

- What level or levels of care are offered?
- Are there any special restrictions? (Some nursing homes do not accept patients with dementia.)
- What programs and services are offered?
- What is the fee? What does the fee include?
- Is there a waiting list? If so, how long is it?
- Is there an initial deposit or down payment required, and if so, what is it?

Q: **Are there any questions to ask specific to the care of a person with dementia?**

A: You should ask:

- Is there an extra charge for care of dementia patients?
- Is there a separate unit or program for people with dementia?
- Are staff members trained or experienced in caring for people with dementia?
- What is the facility's policy on physical restraints?

- What is the facility's policy about using medications to manage the behavior of residents with dementia?
- What provisions are there for assuring the safety of residents who wander? (Remember our discussion in Chapter 7 of locks and alarms.)
- Are there any circumstances under which a resident may be asked to move out of the facility? If so, what are they?

Q: Some of those questions have me worried. Are there really nursing homes that use restraints and medications to manage behavior?

A: Unfortunately, yes. Although the 1989 Federal Nursing Home Reform Law mandated a reduction in the use of restraints, Congress's Office of Technology Assessment reported in 1992 that chemical and physical restraints "are used extensively in nursing homes and are more likely to be used for residents with dementia." They are generally used to control agitated behavior and wandering. But as we have seen, some of the medications used to manage these behaviors have side effects that may actually exacerbate agitation and other symptoms of dementia. Physical restraint may increase agitation, too.

Q: Tell me more about this law. Does it also cover eviction? Are long-term-care facilities allowed to evict someone just because she's difficult to handle?

A: No. The 1989 Federal Nursing Home Reform Law prohibits nursing homes from discharging hard-to-handle residents unless they are a danger to themselves or others. The law requires nursing homes to make an effort to change their practices and meet the residents' needs before evicting them. And if a nursing home does decide to evict a resident, it is required to provide the family with a 30-day written notice. But dumping and arbitrary transfers to mental institutions are still common, according to "Final Indignities," a 1995 investigation conducted by reporters for Newhouse News Service and Maturity News Service.

Q: Is there anything my family can do to prevent this from happening?

A: For starters, make yourself aware of your rights under the law. Nursing homes are not allowed to make threats or force you to remove your loved one from the facility immediately. They must provide you with written notice 30 days before they discharge your loved one. And you have the right to appeal any transfer. You can report violations of this law to your state's long-term-care ombudsman. (Look in the blue pages of your telephone directory for this office or call the local office of the agency on aging.)

Q: Why do some long-term-care facilities resort to such tactics?

A: Primarily because they know very little about how to effectively care for people with dementia. As you know, wandering, calling out, pacing and other agitated behaviors can be frustrating. They can be even more frustrating to people who don't understand them or know how to deal with them. And, according to an article in the October 1994 *Nursing Homes and Senior Citizen Care,* nursing-home staff tend to have an inadequate and inconsistent understanding of dementing illnesses. "Staff have a tendency to relate to residents in ways that tend to increase agitation or increase problem behaviors," in the words of the article. This is beginning to change as the number of people with dementia increases and the need for staff training is emphasized. Still, the problem exists and you need to be aware of it as you go through the process of selecting a facility.

Q: So there are good facilities out there?

A: There certainly are.

Q: How can I find them?

A: When you are touring and investigating facilities, look for those in which staff members are familiar with dementia and treat residents with dementia with respect. (The questions we detailed earlier should help you ferret out this information.) Are residents with dementia tucked out of sight or unable to interact with others, or are they encouraged to interact and socialize? Are they locked into facility-wide routines, or is their routine tailored to suit their needs?

Also ask if residents with dementia are given help and assistance as needed, if a variety of activities are available for them and if those activities vary in ability level.

Q: Wait a minute! Why shouldn't I just look for a facility that offers a special dementia unit or dementia program?

A: Because not all special dementia units and special programs for people with dementia are that special. Some provide exactly the type of care you're looking for; others, however, offer very little except higher prices. They may simply put locks or alarms on a wing of their building and house all residents with dementia in that wing. This may reduce distractions to other residents and prevent those with dementia from leaving the building, but it does little to address their other needs.

In fact, the National Institutes of Health 1991 National Survey of Special Care Units found that only 600 of the 1,500 special-care units surveyed that year offered all six characteristics that should distinguish a special unit.

Q: And what are those six characteristics?

A: So glad you asked. Here they are:

- secured areas
- specially trained staff

- separate dining and activity spaces on the unit
- activity programs designed for people with dementia
- a designated coordinator of such programs
- a process for assessing new patients' needs

Q: **I guess I should ask about those things when I look at facilities with special-care units, shouldn't I?**

A: Yes. But remember that even facilities without special-care units can provide excellent care for people with dementia—through special programs designed specifically for residents with dementia or through customized, individualized care.

Q: **So what should I be looking for?**

A: You want to find a facility that gives people with dementia individual attention, that breaks down tasks for dementia patients so they can succeed, that provides purposeful, appropriate activities, that makes few demands on residents with dementia, and that provides selective access (or egress) or security.

You also want a facility in which staff members are trained in the following:

- causes and types of dementia
- the latest research
- treatment and management strategies
- communication techniques
- behavior-management techniques
- stress-management techniques
- working with families
- psychotropic medications (drugs that affect a person's mental functions or behavior)

Q: What if I find what I believe is a good facility, but staff members haven't had much experience caring for people with dementia?

A: If you believe your loved one will receive the care he needs at the facility, work with the staff. Let them know about your loved one's likes and dislikes and habits. If you know what triggers certain behaviors or you have found effective techniques for managing certain behaviors, let staff members know. There's no need for them to try to reinvent the wheel. Tell staff members what your loved one is capable of doing and what he needs help with. And suggest activities that would be appropriate for him.

Above all, continue to be a major part of his life. Help him adjust, and get help for yourself as well. You, too, have an adjustment to make. We discuss where you can find help in the final chapter.

9 FOR THE CAREGIVING FAMILY

Q: It seems as though the lives of family members can be affected by dementia almost as much as the lives of those with dementia. Am I right?

A: Yes. Dementia affects every member of the family in some way. It prompts strong emotional reactions, affects behavior, lifestyle and relationships, and alters family roles. Family members not only must come to grips with the cognitive, emotional and physical decline of their loved one—an emotionally draining experience in itself—but as caregivers, they must also serve as their loved one's major source of emotional, social and physical support.

Q: So is it normal for family members to feel overwhelmed?

A: It certainly is. Feelings of frustration, anger, insecurity, self-pity, helplessness, uncertainty, embarrassment, fear, anxiety, impatience, guilt, resentfulness, loneliness, isolation and sadness are also normal.

Many family members go into denial; they refuse to believe a problem exists, refuse to believe the diagnosis or believe unrealistically that their loved one will get better. And family members who have accepted the diagnosis may feel sorry for themselves or angry at their situation. As their loved one's dementia progresses and new impairments develop, they may grieve for the loss of their loved one as he used to be.

Feelings of inadequacy may arise when they assume caregiving roles. They may feel insecure about their own abilities and uncertain about the future. They may find themselves so wrapped up in caring for their loved one that they cut themselves off from their normal social lives and end up feeling lonely and isolated.

And when they do take some time for themselves or reflect on their negative feelings, they may feel guilty. This is all perfectly normal. After all, their lives and the life of their loved one have changed in a manner over which they've had little or no control, additional changes are bound to occur, and the end may be a long way off.

Q: What aspect of dementia is hardest for family members to deal with?

A: That depends on the family, its situation and the situation of the person with dementia. Changes in the personality of their loved one or changes in the family's role or lifestyle are difficult for some. For others the hardest adjustment comes with having new—and sometimes extensive—caregiving responsibilities.

DEALING WITH CHANGES

Q: How can family members deal with changes in their loved one's personality?

A: Primarily by learning to accept those changes. Although family members naturally want their loved one to return to the way she was, they must accept her the way she is.

Family members need to realize that the changes are the result of an illness, and that the behavior problems that result are not deliberate attempts to "act out."

Family members also need to be aware that some personality changes may be for the better. Frena Gray Davidson, director of Self-Help Alzheimer's Caregivers Training and Information, a non-profit Alzheimer's education organization, says in her book *The Alzheimer's Sourcebook for Caregivers: A Practical Guide for Getting Through the Day* that some people with Alzheimer's disease retain special abilities, continue to enjoy simple pleasures and may become more open emotionally.

Q: How can families deal with the changes in family roles and lifestyles?

A: Again, primarily by learning to accept them. This can be difficult for both the family and the person with dementia, and it may take time.

It *is* difficult for a spouse to change from partner to caregiver; it *is* difficult for an adult son or daughter to suddenly be responsible for caring for a parent; and it is difficult for a parent to accept care from a child.

Likewise, it is difficult for the family breadwinner to accept being unable to work or a nonworking spouse to suddenly enter the workforce. Giving up or assuming new household roles, too, can be difficult. The family's former financial manager, for example, may feel useless when the books are transferred to another family member. And that family member may be overwhelmed by the financial responsibilities.

All of these changes require adjustment; some require education and training, and all may be made a little easier with the help of counseling and support groups. Education and counseling also make it easier for family members to assume caregiving responsibilities.

DEALING WITH CAREGIVING RESPONSIBILITIES

Q: What type of education do family members need to be effective caregivers?

A: Primarily the type of self-education we've already covered in previous chapters: They need to learn as much as possible about their loved one's disease and about taking care of a person with dementia. Finally, family members need to learn what resources are available to them.

In addition, family caregivers need to learn to take care of themselves. Caregiving is stressful. Studies of caregivers have found increases in new cases of hypertension, depression and heart attack. And yet, as you know, it is vitally important for caregivers to remain healthy if they are to remain able to care for their loved ones.

Q: What type of health-related problems should family caregivers look out for in themselves?

A: Family members need to be alert not only to their overall health, but also for signs of depression and stress.

Signs of depression include:

- sadness or depressed mood
- diminished interest in activities
- weight loss or weight gain
- insomnia
- a slowing or speeding up of activities and mental processes
- fatigue
- feelings of worthlessness or guilt
- difficulty concentrating or thinking
- recurrent thoughts of suicide

Signs of stress include:

- muscle tension
- backaches
- headaches
- sleeping difficulties
- digestive problems
- restlessness
- mood swings
- social withdrawal
- anxiety about the future
- exhaustion
- irritability

Q: What should family members do when they recognize these symptoms in themselves?

A: For starters, they should seek medical or psychological help. Depression can be treated, and medical attention can indicate whether they are experiencing any stress-related health problems. In addition, they can work on ways to reduce the stress in their lives. They can, for example, make sure they're exercising, eating right, getting enough sleep and practicing relaxation techniques. They can also look for extra help, take advantage of respite care and investigate the counseling and support services available to them.

Q: You've mentioned counseling and support services several times. What type of services are available for families and caregivers?

A: In addition to psychiatrists (physicians who specialize in the diagnosis and treatment of mental and psychiatric disorders), the mental-health professionals are:

- psychologists, who are educated in graduate schools of psychology and generally are Ph.D.'s. (Typically a psychologist someone would see for depression would have a subspecialty in clinical or counseling psychology and would be licensed or certified by the state.)

- clinical social workers, who have usually taken a two-year graduate program, including fieldwork, to obtain an M.S.W. (master's in social work). (Most states now license or certify social workers as independent professionals.)

- family therapists, who are specifically trained and licensed in marital and family therapy, and generally have a master's degree in marriage, family and child counseling. (Increasingly states are licensing this as a separate specialty; however, psychiatrists, psychologists and clinical social workers also can offer this type of therapy.)

Also, some members of the clergy are trained to detect depression and, at the very least, to provide referrals to experts.

Q: Are there any other avenues of help and support available?

A: In addition to individual or group counseling from any of the mental-health professionals mentioned, family members may also benefit from participation in one or more support groups. Support groups for family members (and for the ill people themselves) are available for a variety of illnesses, including Alzheimer's disease, Parkinson's disease and stroke.

Further, some support groups are specifically designed for adult children of aging parents and for caregivers. To find a support group, consult the blue pages of your telephone directory or see the Informational and Mutual-Aid Groups section at the back of this book.

Q: **What exactly do support groups do?**

A: Support groups provide education and support to their members. They can be either closed ended—lasting for a set amount of time and covering a certain curriculum—or open ended—lasting indefinitely and providing education, support and interaction with others. They can be led by health-care or caregiving professionals, by people suffering from illness or their caregivers, or by a combination of the two.

Support groups can be an excellent source of information about dementing illnesses, caregiving techniques and available resources. They can also provide a needed social outlet that can help break down the isolation and loneliness that often accompany caregiving.

Q: **To sum up, do you have any general advice to help family members deal with their loved one's illness and their own caregiving responsibilities?**

A: Certainly. To deal with their loved one's illness, family members need to:

- Learn about the loved one's illness.
- Realize that dementia affects the entire family, not just the person with the disease.
- Take responsibility for monitoring their loved one's physical and emotional health.
- Act as advocates for their loved one.
- Communicate with each other.

- Take things one at a time.
- Prepare for the future.

To deal with caregiving responsibilities, they need to:

- Let others help, distribute chores and share the burden.
- Learn about and use the resources available to them.
- Take advantage of respite services.
- Listen to their own feelings.
- Find someone to listen to them.
- Set reasonable goals.
- Live one day at a time.
- Get regular checkups.
- Be alert to signs of depression or stress.
- Exercise, eat right and get enough sleep.
- Make time for themselves.
- Maintain hobbies or find other outlets for venting frustration.
- Maintain a sense of humor.
- Seek counseling and support when needed.

INFORMATIONAL AND MUTUAL-AID GROUPS

Alzheimer's Association
919 N. Michigan Ave., Suite 1000
Chicago, IL 60611-1676
312-335-8700
800-272-3900

> *Provides information and support to family members of people with Alzheimer's disease and related disorders; promotes and funds research; advocates legislation to help those affected by Alzheimer's disease and related disorders; operates the Safe Return and National Respite Care programs; publishes educational brochures, books and a quarterly newsletter; provides support services, including support groups, adult day-care programs, respite-care programs; offers referrals to local chapters.*

Alzheimer's Disease Education and Referral Center
P.O. Box 8250
Silver Spring, MD 20907-8250
301-495-3311
800-438-4380

> *A service of the National Institute on Aging. Provides information on Alzheimer's disease to the general public and health-care professionals; provides publications; offers referrals to agencies and organizations that offer support services.*

American Heart Association
Stroke Connection
7272 Greenville Ave.
Dallas, TX 75231
800-553-6321

> *Provides information and referrals; maintains support-group information; offers peer counseling to stroke survivors and caregivers; publishes* Stroke Connection *magazine.*

American Parkinson's Disease Association
1250 Hylan Blvd., Suite 4B
Staten Island, NY 10305
800-223-2732

> *Provides information about Parkinson's disease and referrals for physicians and support groups.*

Children of Aging Parents
1609 Woodbourne Rd., Suite 302A
Levittown, PA 19057-1511
215-945-6900

> *Provides information and referrals to caregivers of the elderly; assists in starting support groups; publishes bimonthly newsletter. Annual family membership, $20.*

Choice in Dying, Inc.
200 Varick St.
New York, NY 10014-4810
212-366-5540

> *Provides information about state-specific advance directives, counseling about end-of-life decision-making and low-cost educational materials about end-of-life care.*

Elder Care Locator
800-677-1116

> *A public service of the U.S. Department of Health and Human Services' Administration on Aging. Helps people locate local services and resources for senior citizens.*

Huntington's Disease Society of America
140 W. 22nd St.
New York, NY 10011
212-242-1968
800-345-4372

> *Provides information on Huntington's disease; offers referrals to local chapters and support services.*

Joint Commission on Accreditation of Healthcare Organizations
1 Renaissance Blvd.
Oakbrook Terrace, IL 60181
708-916-5600

> *Accredits home health agencies and long-term-care facilities.*

Multiple Sclerosis Association of America
601 White Horse Pike
Oaklyn, NJ 08107
800-833-4672

Provides information on multiple sclerosis; offers peer counseling; loans equipment; publishes bimonthly newsletter.

National Family Caregivers Association
9621 E. Bexhill Dr.
Kensington, MD 20895-3104
301-942-6430
800-896-3650

Provides information, education and support to family caregivers; operates an information clearinghouse; provides educational materials and speakers; advocates respite care; publishes quarterly newsletter. Membership, $15.

National League for Nursing
350 Hudson St.
New York, NY 10014
212-989-9393

Accredits home health agencies.

National Meals on Wheels Foundation
2675 44th St. S.W., Suite 305
Grand Rapids, MI 49509
800-999-6262
616-531-9909

Provides information on Meals on Wheels program; offers referrals to local chapters.

National Multiple Sclerosis Society
733 Third Ave.
New York, NY 10017-3288
800-344-4867

Provides information about multiple sclerosis; offers referrals to local chapters; publishes Inside M.S. *three times annually.*

National Organization for Rare Disorders
100 Route 37
P.O. Box 8923
New Fairfield, CT 06812-8923
203-746-6518
800-447-6673

Provides information and networking for people with rare disorders.

National Parkinson Foundation
1501 N.W. 9th Ave.
Bob Hope Road
Miami, FL 33136
800-327-4545

Conducts research on Parkinson's disease; provides information on Parkinson's disease; offers referrals to physicians in the United States and Europe; publishes Parkinson's Quarterly Report.

National Stroke Association
8480 E. Orchard Rd., Suite 1000
Englewood, CO 80111-5015
303-771-1700
800-STROKE (787-6537)

Provides information on strokes; offers counseling and assistance; offers referrals to organizations establishing stroke programs and support groups; provides materials on stroke prevention, treatment and care; sells publications and videos; publishes the Journal of Stroke and Cerebrovascular Disease *and the* Be Stroke Smart *newsletter. Individual memberships ($20) include a newsletter subscription and a discount on publications.*

Parkinson's Disease Foundation
William Black Memorial Research Building
Columbia-Presbyterian Medical Center
650-710 W. 168th St.
New York, NY 10032
212-923-4700
800-457-6676

Conducts research on and provides information about Parkinson's disease; offers counseling; has clinical specialist on call to answer questions; provides list of support groups; publishes newsletter.

Visiting Nurse Associations of America
3801 E. Florida Ave., Suite 900
Denver, CO 80210
800-426-2547
303-753-0218

> *Provides referrals to local Visiting Nurse Associations around the country.*

Well Spouse Foundation
610 Lexington Ave., Suite 814
New York, NY 10022
212-644-1241
800-838-0879

> *Offers support to spouses and partners of chronically ill or disabled individuals; provides referrals to existing local support groups; aids in establishing local support groups; publishes bimonthly newsletter.*

Wilson's Disease Association
P.O. Box 75324
Washington, DC 20013
703-743-1415

> *Provides information on Wilson's disease; offers support to people with Wilson's disease and their families and friends; publishes semiannual newsletter.*

GLOSSARY

Acetylcholine: A neurotransmitter; a substance that allows messages to travel from one nerve to another. Acetylcholine is deficient in people with Alzheimer's disease.

Acetylcholinesterase: An enzyme that breaks down acetylcholine.

Activities of daily living: Normal everyday actions, such as eating, drinking, dressing and grooming.

Adult day care: Service that provides older adults with supervised care, activities and companionship during set hours of the day.

Advance directive: Written document that, in the case of a serious illness, either clarifies an individual's wishes for health care or names a person to make health-care decisions for that individual if he or she is unable to do so.

Agenda behavior: A behavior with a specific goal or purpose.

Agnosia: Inability to recognize familiar objects or to associate an object with its use.

AIDS (acquired immune deficiency syndrome): Disease of the immune system caused by infection with the human immunodeficiency virus (HIV).

AIDS dementia complex: Dementia that occurs when the human immunodeficiency virus (HIV) infects the central nervous system.

Allele: One of two or more possible forms of a gene.

Alzheimer's disease: A progressive, degenerative brain disease that impairs memory, thinking and behavior.

Amyloid precursor protein (APP): A protein that, when broken down in an abnormal way, creates beta amyloid.

Antianxiety medications: Minor tranquilizers; used to treat some symptoms of dementia.

Anticholinergic drugs: Drugs that counteract the activity of the neurotransmitter acetylcholine.

Anticoagulant: A drug that helps prevent or delay blood clots; a *blood thinner.*

Antidepressants: Drugs used to treat depression.

Antipsychotics: Also known as *major tranquilizers* or *neuroleptics;* drugs given to lessen the symptoms of a severe mental illness; used to treat some symptoms of dementia.

Apolipoprotein E (ApoE): A substance that plays a role in the movement and distribution of cholesterol for repairing nerve cells.

Apraxia: Inability to voluntarily perform skilled movements.

Assisted living facility: Long-term-care facility that offers custodial care.

Atherosclerosis: Condition in which the inner layers of the artery walls become thick and irregular due to deposits of fat, cholesterol and other substances.

Autosomal dominant: Pattern of inheritance in which a dominant gene on a non-sex-determining chromosome makes a certain characteristic.

Benign senescent forgetfulness: Minor degree of forgetfulness that occurs normally with age.

Beta amyloid: Sticky protein that appears when amyloid precursor protein is broken down in an abnormal way; comprises the neuritic plaques in the brains of people with Alzheimer's disease.

Binswanger's disease: A form of vascular dementia in which hypertension or atherosclerosis produces infarcts in small blood vessels deep in the brain.

Calcium channel blockers: Drugs that prevent calcium from entering cells.

Catastrophic reaction: An emotionally violent response to a relatively insignificant incident.

Cerebral cortex: Area of the brain that controls higher mental functions, general movement and behavioral reactions.

Cerebral embolism: Clot or other material that originates somewhere in the body, travels through the bloodstream and lodges in and blocks an artery supplying the brain.

Cerebrospinal fluid (CSF): Fluid that flows around and protects the brain and spinal canal; examination of CSF can help diagnose diseases of the central nervous system.

Choline acetyltransferase: Enzyme needed to make acetylcholine.

Cholinergic drugs: Drugs that stimulate the cholinergic system.

Cholinergic system: System of nerves that communicate with the help of the neurotransmitter acetylcholine.

Circumlocution: A form of language dysfunction in which a person talks around a word, using descriptions rather than the word itself.

Computerized axial tomography (CAT): See **Computerized tomography (CT).**

Computerized tomography (CT): A computer-enhanced series of cross-sectional x-ray images of selected parts of the body. Also called *computerized axial tomography (CAT).*

Congestive heart failure: A condition in which the heart fails to pump blood effectively.

Corticosteroid: Also known as steroids; hormones made in the outer layer of the adrenal gland; often prescribed to prevent swelling or reduce allergic reactions.

Creutzfeldt-Jakob disease: Rare, fatal brain disease, caused by an unknown organism—possibly a virus—that causes dementia and a variety of other neurological symptoms.

Custodial care: Nonmedical, long-term care; room, board and personal services.

Decubitus ulcer: Bedsore, pressure ulcer; a swollen sore or ulcer of the skin over a bony part of the body resulting from prolonged pressure.

Delusion: A belief or perception held as true by a person, even though it is not.

Dementia: A syndrome in which mental functions deteriorate; it includes the impairment of more than one cognitive, or intellectual, ability, is persistent and is severe enough to interfere with a person's daily functioning. More than 70 diseases, disorders and conditions can cause dementia.

Deprenyl: A monoamine oxidase inhibitor with antioxidant properties; used to slow the progression of Parkinson's disease and being studied as a possible treatment for Alzheimer's disease.

Depression: Persistent feelings of sadness, despair and discouragement, which may be a symptom of an underlying mental or physical disorder.

Diuretics: Drugs that promote urination, thus speeding the body's elimination of sodium and water; often used to control blood pressure.

Dopamine: A neurotransmitter in the brain thought to be associated with depression and Parkinson's disease.

Drug intoxication: Adverse reaction to a drug or drugs.

Durable power of attorney for health care: Legal document that transfers health-care decision-making power to a designated representative in the event that a person becomes unable to make his or her own health-care decisions.

Echolalia: Meaningless repetition of another's words or phrases.

Electrocardiogram (EKG): A graphic record of electrical impulses produced by the heart.

Electroconvulsive therapy: A treatment for depression in which low-voltage electric current is sent to the brain to induce a convulsion or seizure.

Electroencephalography (EEG): Diagnostic test in which electrodes are put on the scalp to pick up electrical impulses transmitted and received by the brain cells.

Emotional lability: Unstable emotions.

Flatness of affect: Apathy; lacking emotion.

Frontal lobe: Part of the brain that influences personality and is linked to higher mental activities, such as planning and judgment.

Geriatrician: Doctor who specializes in dealing with the diseases of the elderly and the problems associated with aging.

Guardian: A person or institution granted, by the court, legal responsibility for another person and authority to manage that person's affairs.

Hallucinations: Sensual perceptions of things that do not exist.

Hematoma: A collection of blood that has escaped from the vessels and become trapped in the tissues of the skin or in an organ.

Hippocampus: Lower region of the brain; controls emotions.

Home attendant: See **Personal-care aide.**

Home health agency: An organization that provides health care in the home.

Home health aide: A worker who assists in providing health- and personal-care services to a patient living at home.

Huntington's chorea: See **Huntington's disease.**

Huntington's disease: Rare, inherited disease characterized by progressive dementia and irregular, involuntary movements of the limbs and facial muscles.

Hydergine: Nootropic drug used to treat vascular dementia and Alzheimer's disease.

Hydrocephalus: Condition in which there is an abnormal amount of cerebrospinal fluid, often under high pressure, in the brain.

Hypertension: A chronic increase in blood pressure above its normal range—generally systolic readings greater than 140 and/or diastolic readings greater than 90 over a period of time.

Hypoglycemia: Condition caused by low amount of sugar in the blood; may result in dementia symptoms.

Hypothyroidism: Reduced thyroid function; a condition that may produce dementia symptoms.

Hypoxia: A deficiency of oxygen in the body's cells.

Indomethacin: A nonsteroidal anti-inflammatory drug being tested as a possible treatment for Alzheimer's disease.

Infarct: Area of tissue that is dead or dying, having been deprived of blood.

Intermediate care facility: Nursing home that provides health care and services to people who do not require the care and services of a hospital or skilled nursing facility.

Lacunar state: Form of vascular dementia generally caused by the effects of hypertension on the small blood vessels deep in the brain.

Lewy bodies: Protein deposits that appear in the deteriorating brain neurons of people with Lewy body dementia.

Lewy body dementia: Rare, degenerative brain disease of unknown origin that causes dementia.

Living will: Legal document that describes what types of medical treatments a person will permit in order to prolong his or her life.

Lumbar puncture: A sampling of cerebrospinal fluid removed from the spinal canal by means of a long needle; used to diagnose diseases of and injuries to the brain and spinal cord.

Magnetic resonance imaging (MRI): A diagnostic technique that provides high-quality cross-sectional images of organs and structures in the body using a magnetic field (instead of radiation).

Meningitis: Inflammation or swelling of the membranes covering the brain and spinal cord.

Mixed dementia: A combination of Alzheimer's disease and vascular dementia.

Multi-infarct dementia: The most common form of vascular dementia; caused by a series of small strokes that leave areas of dead brain cells known as infarcts.

Multiple sclerosis: Disease of the central nervous system in which the protective myelin covering of nerve fibers of the brain and spinal cord is gradually lost; its symptoms include problems with movement and coordination, sensory problems, vision problems, urinary incontinence, problems with mental functioning, lack of energy and fatigue.

Myelin: Fatty substance that covers and protects nerve fibers.

Nerve growth factor (NGF): Hormone that affects the growth and care of nerve cells.

Neuritic plaques: Deposits of beta amyloid and the debris of dying neurons found in the brains of people with Alzheimer's disease.

Neurofibrillary tangles: Twisted nerve-cell fibers that appear inside neurons in the brains of people with Alzheimer's disease.

Neuroleptics: Antipsychotic medications; major tranquilizers.

Neurologist: Doctor who specializes in the brain and nervous system.

Neuron: Nerve cell.

Neuropsychological testing: Neurological tests and standardized intelligence tests designed to help determine whether changes in mental status or performance are caused by aging or a disease.

Neurosyphilis: Infection of the central nervous system caused by the bacterium that causes syphilis; occurs in the third, final stage of syphilis and was once a common cause of dementia.

Neurotransmitter: A chemical that assists in sending signals among nerve cells in the brain.

NMDA receptors: Drugs that block the receptors responsible for calcium secretion in the brain; being studied as a treatment for AIDS dementia complex.

Nonsteroidal anti-inflammatory drugs: Drugs used to reduce inflammation that are not based on steroids.

Nootropic: A drug whose mechanisms experts do not understand.

Normal-pressure hydrocephalus: Form of hydrocephalus in which the pressure of the cerebrospinal fluid remains normal; a cause of dementia.

Paid companion: A person hired to act as a companion to another person.

Parkinson's disease: Progressive disorder of the central nervous system that causes a deficiency of the neurotransmitter dopamine; its symptoms include tremors, stiffness in the limbs and joints, speech impediments, difficulty initiating physical movement and dementia.

Personal-care aide: Worker who provides services that help a person meet the demands of daily living.

Pharmacotherapy: The use of pharmacological agents in the treatment of mental disorders.

Physostigmine: A drug that inhibits acetylcholinesterase; being studied for the treatment of Alzheimer's disease.

Pick bodies: Spherical deposits of protein that appear in the neurons of people with Pick's disease.

Pick's disease: Progressive, degenerative disease that affects the front part of the brain, causing dementia.

Platelet inhibitors: Drugs that prevent platelets from collecting; *blood thinners.*

Positron emission tomography (PET): A technique for making computer-generated images of the brain or other body organs by means of radioactive isotopes injected into the body.

Power of attorney: Legal document that permits a second person to make all legal decisions for another person.

Prednisone: A steroid used to treat severe swelling and to stop the body from having an immune response to an allergy-causing substance; being tested as a possible treatment for Alzheimer's disease.

Presenile dementia: Dementia occurring in a person below the age of 65.

Psychomotor retardation: Excessively slow or sluggish motor actions directly proceeding from decreasing mental activity.

Psychotherapy: Therapy employing psychological methods; used to treat depression.

Radioactive isotopes: Unstable forms of an element, which give off radiation as the nuclei of their atoms decay; used in certain imaging techniques.

Residential care home: Long-term-care facility that offers custodial care.

Respite care: Temporary care for a person whose care or supervision is normally provided by a family member at home; respite care gives family members temporary relief from care-giving demands.

Senile: Characteristic of old age or the process of aging; often used to mean forgetful.

Senile dementia: Dementia occurring in a person 65 or older.

Senile dementia of the Alzheimer's type: Alzheimer's disease or a similar dementia occurring in a person 65 or older.

Senility: The state of being senile; often used to mean forgetfulness.

Single photon emission computed tomography (SPECT): A technique for making computer-generated images of the brain or other organs by means of radioactive isotopes injected into the body.

Sitter: A person hired to stay with and supervise another person.

Skilled nursing facility: A nursing home that provides skilled nursing care and related services for seriously ill patients who require inpatient medical or nursing care similar to that received in a hospital.

Strategic infarct: Form of vascular dementia caused by small infarcts strategically positioned in blood vessels that serve areas of the brain that control several cognitive processes.

Stroke: Sudden loss of function of part of the brain due to an interference in blood supply.

Subdural hematoma: Hematoma, or pool of blood, between the brain and one of its protective membranes.

Sundowning: Agitation and restlessness in the late afternoon or early evening.

Syndrome: A collection of signs and symptoms indicative of an illness or disorder.

Tacrine: Also known as *tetrahydroaminoacridine,* the only drug currently approved to treat Alzheimer's disease. Tacrine improves cognitive abilities, such as memory and learning, by stopping acetylcholinesterase, an enzyme, from breaking down acetylcholine.

Tau: A protein found in the neurofibrillary tangles in the brains of people with Alzheimer's disease.

Temporal lobe: Outer lower region of the brain; associated with memory and learning.

Ticlopidine: A platelet inhibitor used to prevent and treat stroke.

Tropicamide: Drug that dilates the pupil of the eye; being studied for its possible use in diagnosing Alzheimer's disease.

Trust: Legal directive that enables one or more persons or institutions to be named to manage the property, assets or other financial matters of another person.

Tuberculosis: A long-term infection caused by a bacterium; a cause of meningitis.

Vascular dementia: Dementia caused by problems with the blood vessels, or vascular system.

Vasculitis: Swelling of the blood vessels caused by systemic diseases or allergic reactions.

Vasodilators: Drug used to dilate, or widen, blood vessels.

Wernicke-Korsakoff syndrome: Syndrome characterized by incoordination, memory loss, confusion, apathy and drowsiness; caused by a deficiency of thiamine brought on by prolonged alcohol abuse.

Wilson's disease: Rare, inherited disorder in which copper accumulates in the liver and is then released and taken up into other parts of the body; can cause hepatitis, cirrhosis, kidney problems, tremors, muscle rigidity, speech problems and dementia.

Zidovudine: Drug used to treat AIDS; also called AZT.

SUGGESTED READING

Aronson, Miriam K., Ed.D., ed. *Understanding Alzheimer's Disease.* New York: Charles Scribner's Sons, Macmillan Publishing Co., 1988. A publication of the Alzheimer's Disease and Related Disorders Association.

Bair, Frank E., ed. *Alzheimer's, Stroke and 29 Other Neurological Disorders Sourcebook.* Detroit, Mich.: Omnigraphics, Inc., 1993. Health Reference Series, vol. 2. Compiled by the National Institute of Neurological and Communicative Disorders and Stroke.

Carroll, David. *When Your Loved One Has Alzheimer's.* New York: Harper and Row, 1989.

Cohen, Donna, Ph.D., and Carl Eisdorfer, Ph.D., M.D. *The Loss of Self: A Family Resource for the Care of Alzheimer's Disease and Related Disorders.* New York: W.W. Norton and Co., 1986.

Coughlan, Patricia Brown. *Facing Alzheimer's: Family Caregivers Speak.* New York: Ballantine Books, 1993.

Davidson, Frena Gray. *The Alzheimer's Sourcebook for Caregivers: A Practical Guide for Getting Through the Day.* Los Angeles: Lowell House, 1994.

Dippel, Raye Lynn, Ph.D., and J. Thomas Hutton, M.D., Ph.D., ed. *Caring for the Alzheimer Patient: A Practical Guide.* Second edition. Buffalo, NY: Prometheus Books, 1991.

Driscoll, Eileen Higgins. *Alzheimer's: A Handbook for the Caregiver.* Boston: Branden Books, 1994.

Gard, Robert E. *Beyond the Thin Line: A Personal Journey into the World of Alzheimer's Disease.* Madison, Wisc.: Prairie Oak Press, 1992.

Gruetzner, Howard, M.Ed. *Alzheimer's: A Caregiver's Guide and Sourcebook.* New York: John Wiley and Sons Inc., 1992.

Henig, Robin Marantz. *The Myth of Senility: The Truth About the Brain and Aging.* Glenview, Ill.: Scott Foresman and Co., 1988. An AARP publication.

Hodgson, Harriet. *Alzheimer's: Finding the Words: A Communication Guide for Those Who Care.* Minneapolis: Chronimed Publishing, 1995.

Mace, Nancy L., M.A., and Peter V. Rabins, M.D., M.P.H. *The 36-Hour Day: A Family Guide to Caring for Persons with Alzheimer's Disease, Related Dementing Illnesses, and Memory Loss Later in Life.* Rev. ed. Baltimore: Johns Hopkins University Press, 1991.

Markin, R.E.: *The Alzheimer's Cope Book.* New York: Citadel Press, 1992.

Miner, Gary D., Ph.D.; Linda A. Winters-Miner, Ph.D.; John P. Blass, M.D., Ph.D.; Ralph W. Richter, M.D.; and Jimmie L. Valentine, Ph.D. *Caring for Alzheimer's Patients: A Guide for Family and Healthcare Providers.* New York: Insight Books, Plenum Press, 1989.

Powell, Lenore S., Ed.D., and Katie Courtice. *Alzheimer's Disease: A Guide for Families.* Rev. ed. Reading, Mass.: Addison-Wesley Publishing, 1993.

Roach, Marion. *Another Name for Madness.* Boston: Houghton Mifflin Co., 1985.

Safford, Florence, D.S.W. *Caring for the Mentally Impaired Elderly: A Family Guide.* New York: Henry Holt and Co., 1986.

Sheridan, Carmel, M.A. *Failure-Free Activities for the Alzheimer's Patient: A Guidebook for Caregivers.* Oakland, Calif.: Cottage Books, 1987.

INDEX

A

Acetylcholine, 56, 173
Acetylcholinesterase, 88, 173
Acquired immune deficiency
   syndrome (AIDS). *See* AIDS
Activities of daily living, 119-124,
   173
Adrenergic stimulants, 27
Adult day care, 103, 104, 112, 141,
   145-146, 173
Advance directive, 110, 111-112,
   173
Age
   Alzheimer's disease and, 13,
      16-17
   death rates and, 13
   dementia and, 16-17
Agenda behavior, 131, 173
Agitation, 94-96, 134
Agnosia, 19, 173
AIDS, 16, 41, 44-45, 77, 173
AIDS dementia complex, 44-45, 173
Alcohol, 25, 28-30
Aldomet. *See* Methyldopa
Aldoril. *See* Methyldopa/
   hydrochlorothiazide
Allele, 61, 173
Alprazolam, 27, 95-96
Aluminum, 57, 58
Alzheimer Association's Safe Return
   Program, 132
Alzheimer's disease. *See also*
   Dementia
   age and, 13, 16-17
   causes
      cholinergic system deficit, 57

environmental toxins, 57,
   58-59
free radicals, 57, 59, 90, 91
genetics, 57, 60-63, 74
immune system, 57, 59
nerve growth factor (NGF)
   deficit, 57-58, 89, 92
viral or infectious agents, 57,
   58, 73
complications, 13-14
costs, generally, 99-100
defined, 13, 173
dementia vs., 14
depression and, 21
diagnosis, 81-83
early- vs. late onset, 60-61
effects, 13-14, 52-56
familial, 60
incidence, 13, 15
informational and mutual-aid
   groups, 168-172
mechanics, 55-56
prevention
   anti-inflammatory drugs, 64,
      92-93
   education level, 65-66
   estrogen, 64-65
   head trauma, 66
   "use it or lose it" theory, 65
progression, 14
stages, 52-54
support groups, 166
symptoms, generally, 14
treatment, 87-93
Amitriptyline, 27, 96
Amyloid precursor protein (APP),
   56, 60, 174